Pediatric Cataract

Siddharth Agrawal
Editor

Pediatric Cataract

For Every Ophthalmologist

Springer

Editor
Siddharth Agrawal
Department of Ophthalmology
King George's Medical University
Lucknow, UP
India

ISBN 978-981-16-1735-5 ISBN 978-981-16-1736-2 (eBook)
https://doi.org/10.1007/978-981-16-1736-2

This Springer imprint is published by the registered company Springer Nature Singapore Pte Ltd.
The registered company address is: 152 Beach Road, #21-01/04 Gateway East, Singapore 189721, Singapore

Dedicated

to

the hundreds of parents who

have trusted me

with

the eyes of their children

Foreword

Pediatric cataract is among the leading causes of childhood blindness, especially in developing countries like India. Right from examination of these patients, to preoperative planning and intraocular lens calculation, considerations for general anesthesia, and surgical technique including primary posterior capsulotomy, all pose a unique challenge which is unlike adult cataract surgery. The job of a pediatric cataract surgeon does not end with the completion of a successful surgery. Intensive control of postoperative inflammation and monitoring for visual axis opacification/glaucoma are a must. Either of these conditions may require secondary surgical procedures over the course of follow-up. Not surprisingly, most ophthalmologists shy away from management of this condition leading to significant backlog of cases. There is a need to train more cataract surgeons in the management of pediatric cataract to clear this backlog.

This book by Dr. Siddharth Agrawal brings together the approach to pediatric cataract in a very lucid and simplified manner. The initial chapters address the development of the human eye, associated anomalies, and the etio-pathogenesis of cataract in children. The discussion remains clinical to keep the reader interested. The subsequent chapters on preoperative workup and intraocular lenses are about the issues to be addressed prior to the surgery. The chapter on pediatric cataract surgery discusses in detail the modifications required and special procedures to be performed while operating on children. A separate chapter on complications will help the reader to prevent, identify, and manage the usual complications. Traumatic cataracts and their associations have been well explained in the penultimate chapter. The last chapter is on rehabilitation after cataract surgery and includes management of amblyopia which is essential for satisfactory outcomes.

Authored by some of the stalwarts in the field of pediatric cataract surgery, this book is surely a treasure for those stepping into this challenging world. The language is easy to understand, the figures and tables make the reading interesting, and the multiple-choice questions reinforce the important concepts. Having spent over 36 years in the field of pediatric cataract surgery, I am confident that this book will serve as an important resource for both trainee and accomplished surgeons alike.

Jagat Ram
Director, Post Graduate Institute of Medical Education and Research (PGIMER), Chandigarh, India

Professor, Advanced Eye Centre, PGIMER, Chandigarh, India

Preface

Being in a government tertiary care institute of India, I frequently see extremely late presentation of congenital cataract, which compromises its optimal management. What is more disheartening is that while almost each district has numerous qualified and well equipped eye surgeons successfully managing adult cataracts, there are very few handling pediatric cases. Perhaps they are wary of the challenging preoperative workup, the modifications required in surgical technique, and the longer postoperative rehabilitation.

The parents often have to travel across the state or states to reach the nearest center making the treatment unnecessarily delayed and expensive. The waiting list at these centers often runs into months. The delayed management makes the eventual outcome unsatisfactory. The burden of a visually handicapped child on the family and the society cannot be overestimated. More so, when it is preventable by timely intervention.

Just as patients have been the motivation behind this work, practicing ophthalmologists and ophthalmology residents are the intended audience. The aim is to encourage a larger number of ophthalmic surgeons to handle pediatric cataract. Patience, sympathetic attitude, and a slight upgradation in skills are the only requirements. While the discussion across the chapters remains clinical, relevant theoretical concepts have been emphasized to enable clearer understanding. I would appreciate inputs from readers to make future editions more useful.

Dr Rajat Mohan, my colleague and friend has been associated with this work since its inception. He is an excellent clinician and one of the most humane persons that I have known. I am fortunate to have his support. I am thankful to my Head of the Department (HoD) Prof Apjit Kaur for providing the appropriate environment for this work. I express my gratitude to my mentor and former HoD Prof Vinita Singh for all her confidence in me. I'm sure she feels proud of me.

I am extremely grateful to all my co-authors for their time and effort. They have been patient and always responded promptly to all the requests. I am sure they feel satisfied with the final outcome. I look forward to collaborating with each of them in future, as well.

This work has been a great learning exercise for me. It has been stimulating and pleasantly time consuming. Blessings of parents, unconditional support of my wife, encouragement from my brother, and love of my daughters have been the essential ingredients for all my achievements.

I am most thankful to the almighty as He is the actual doer.

Lucknow, India
April 2021

Siddharth Agrawal

Notice

Knowledge and best practice in ophthalmology are ever-changing. Standard safety precautions must be followed, and as research and clinical experience broaden our knowledge, changes in treatment and drug therapy may become necessary. Readers are advised to check the most current product information provided by the manufacturer of each drug to be administered to verify the recommended dose, the method and duration of administration, and contraindications. While using the information provided in this book, it is the responsibility of the treating physician, relying on his experience and knowledge of the patient, to determine the best treatment for each individual patient. Neither the publisher nor the editor or the authors assume any liability for any injury and/or damage to persons or property arising from this publication.

Contents

Editor and Contributors

About the Editor

Siddharth Agrawal, (MS, DNB) has completed his medical education from King George's Medical University (KGMU), Lucknow, India. He has received advanced cataract training at Sankara Nethralaya, Chennai. He is presently Additional Professor of Ophthalmology and in charge of Strabismus and Pediatric Vision Clinic of the department at KGMU. He has many peer-reviewed publications on the subject, is a reviewer for several international journals, and has delivered lectures and conducted instruction courses at various international conferences across the globe including APAO Sydney (2011), ISO Guangzhou (2013), APGC Hong Kong (2014), WOC Tokyo (2014), and APAO Singapore (2017). He has two extramural research grants, has received five international travel fellowships, and has visited SNEC (Singapore) in 2014, Weil Cornell University (New York, USA) in 2015, and Columbia University (New York, USA) in 2018 as observer in the sub-specialty. He has edited and co-authored a textbook on strabismus, has a patent, is co-in-charge of the postgraduate teaching program of the department, and conducts about 200 pediatric cataract surgeries each year.

Contributors

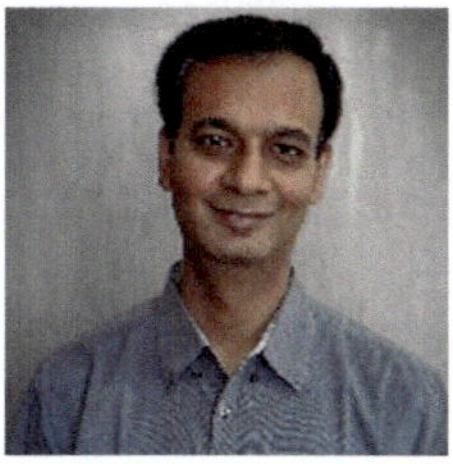

Siddharth Agrawal
Department of Ophthalmology, King George's Medical University, Lucknow, India

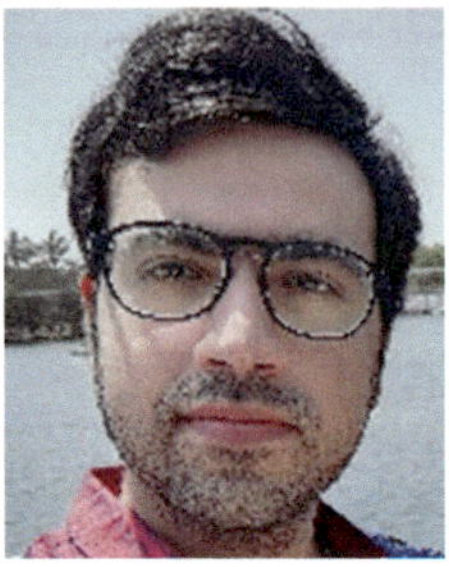

Amber Amar Bhayana
Dr Rajendra Prasad Centre for Ophthalmic Sciences, All India Institute of Medical Sciences (AIIMS), New Delhi, India

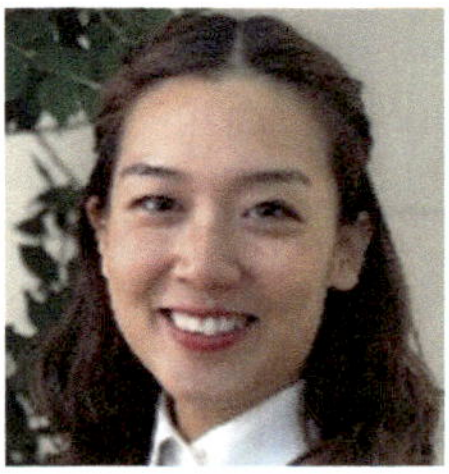

Joyce J. Chan
Moorfields Eye Hospital, London, UK
Department of Ophthalmology and Visual Sciences, The Chinese University of Hong Kong, Hong Kong Eye Hospital, Kowloon, Hong Kong

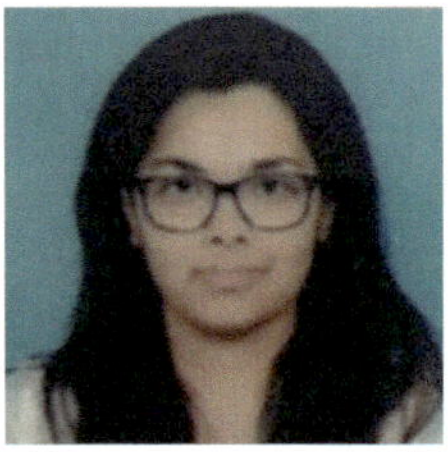

Isha Chaturvedi
Department of Ophthalmology, Sanjay Gandhi Post Graduate Institute of Medical Sciences, Lucknow, India

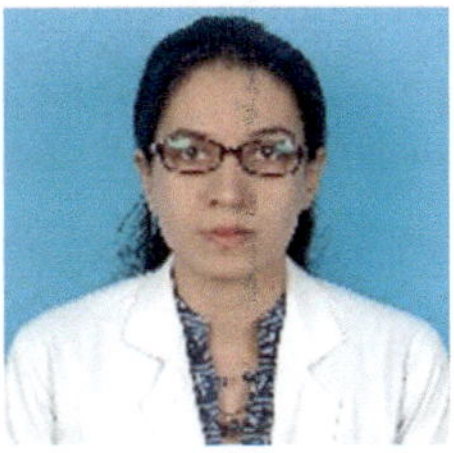

Chirakshi Dhull
Eye Q Hospital, Gurugram, India

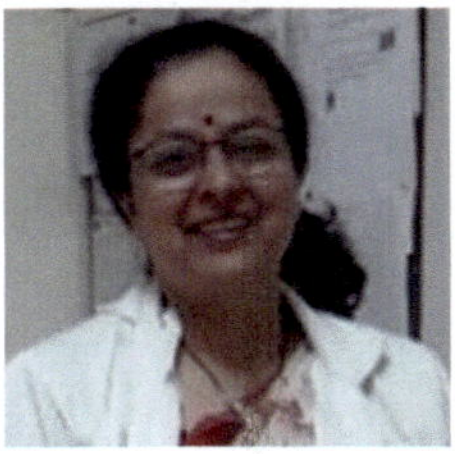

Suma Ganesh
Dr Shroff's Charity Eye Hospital, Delhi, India

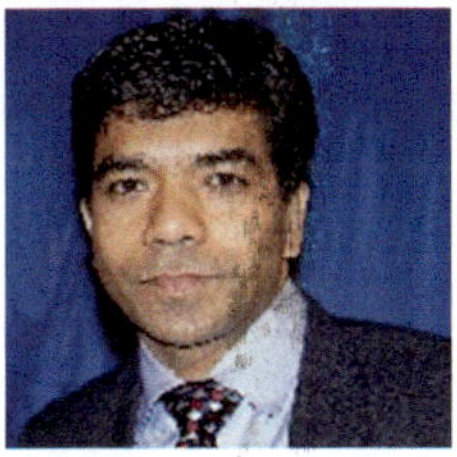

Vikas Kanaujia
Department of Ophthalmology, Sanjay Gandhi Post Graduate Institute of Medical Sciences, Lucknow, India

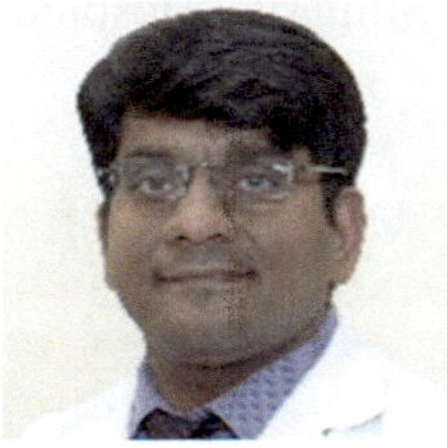

Rajat Kapoor
Child Sight Institute, LV Prasad Eye Institute, Hyderabad, India

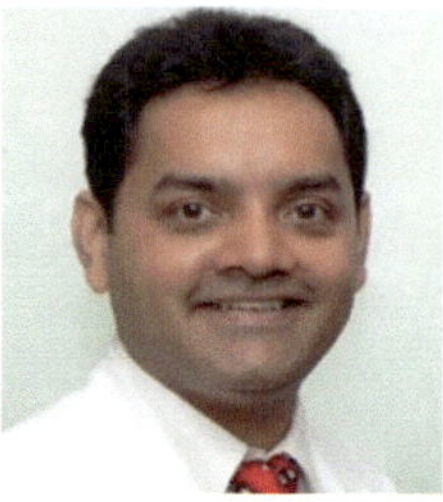

Ramesh Kekunnaya
Child Sight Institute, LV Prasad Eye Institute, Hyderabad, India

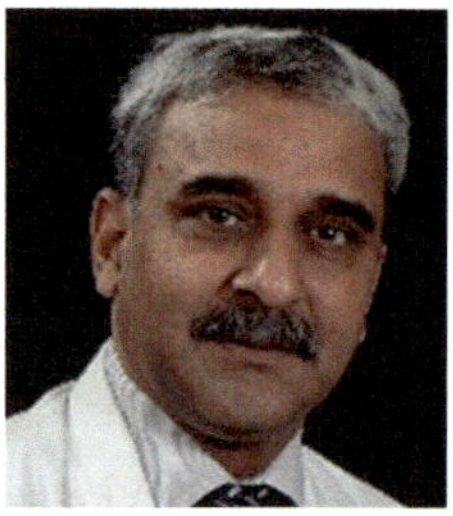

Sudarshan Khokhar
Dr Rajendra Prasad Centre for Ophthalmic Sciences, All India Institute of Medical Sciences (AIIMS), New Delhi, India

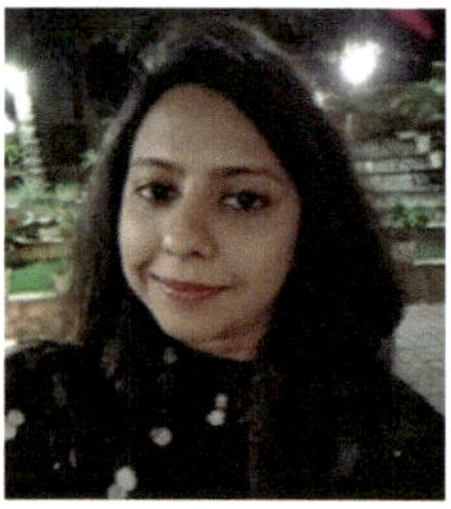

Rolli Khurana
Eye Department, Armed Forces Medical Services, Military Hospital, Ahmedabad, India

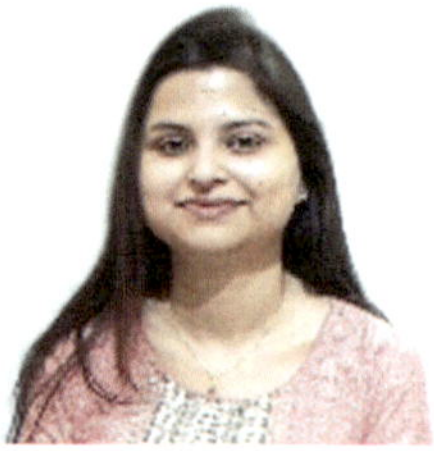

Nitika Pandey
Department of Ophthalmology, King George's Medical University, Lucknow, India

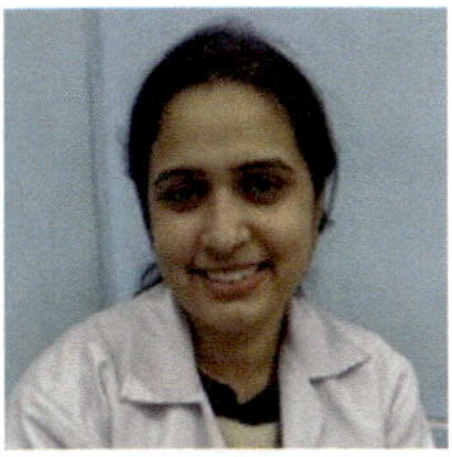

Soveeta Rath
Dr Shroff's Charity Eye Hospital, Delhi, India

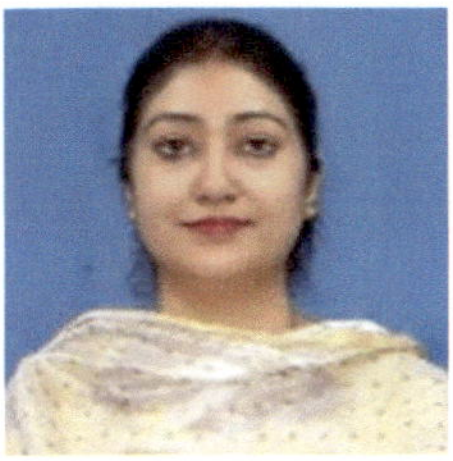

Priya Singh
Department of Ophthalmology, Sanjay Gandhi Post Graduate Institute of Medical Sciences, Lucknow, India

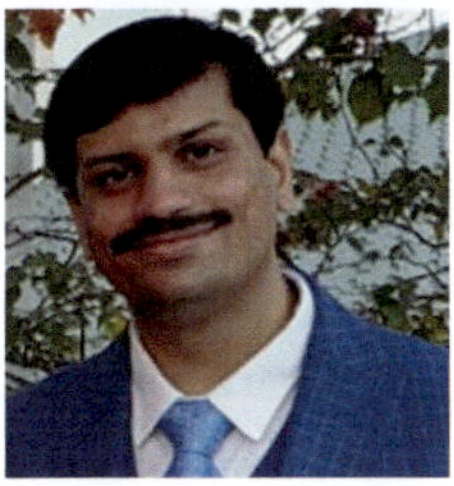

Rajat M. Srivastava
Department of Ophthalmology, King George's Medical University, Lucknow, India

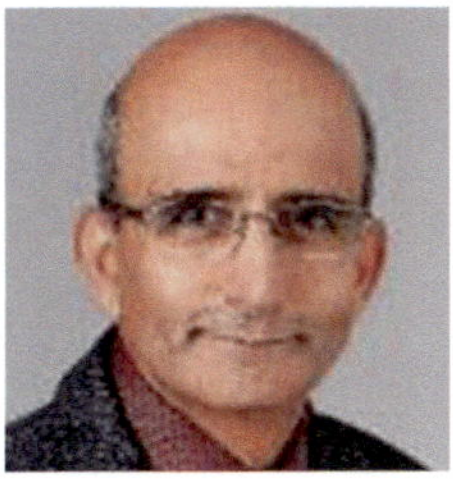

Abhay R. Vasavada
Raghudeep Eye Hospital, Iladevi Cataract & IOL Research Centre, Ahmedabad, India

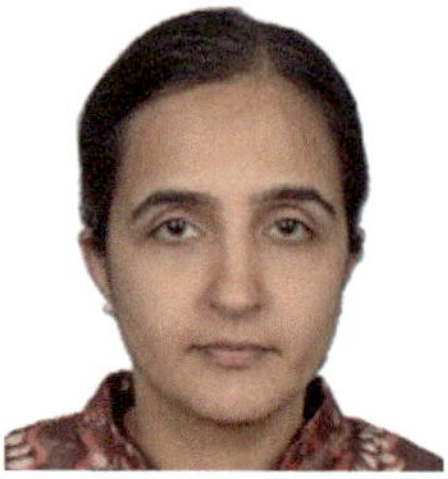

Vaishali Vasavada
Raghudeep Eye Hospital, Iladevi Cataract & IOL Research Centre, Ahmedabad, India

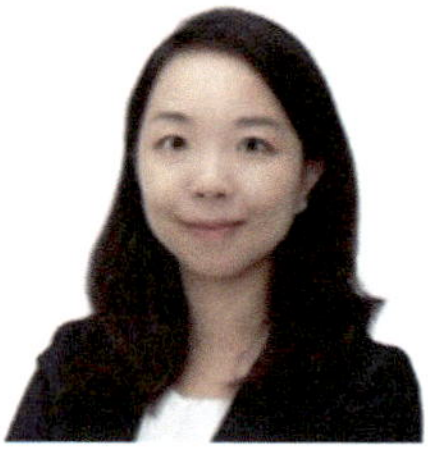

Emily S. Wong
Department of Ophthalmology and Visual Sciences, The Chinese University of Hong Kong, Hong Kong Eye Hospital, Kowloon, Hong Kong

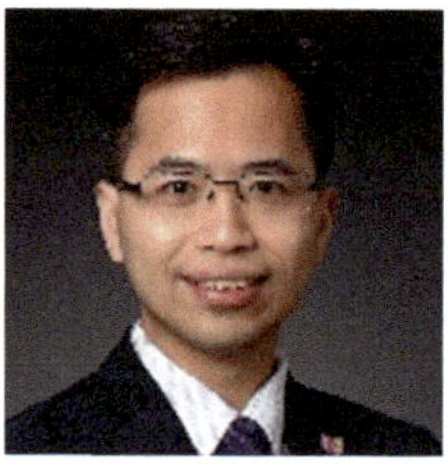

Jason C. Yam
Department of Ophthalmology and Visual Sciences, The Chinese University of Hong Kong, Hong Kong Eye Hospital, Kowloon, Hong Kong

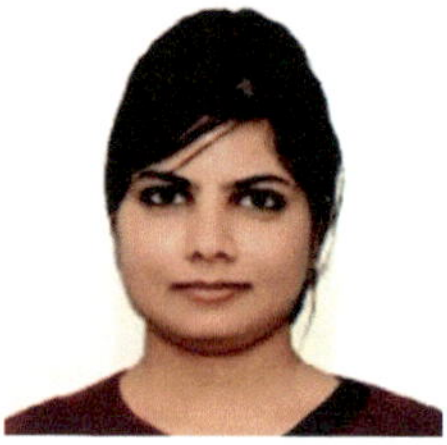

Ankita
Department of Ophthalmology, Ganesh Shankar Vidyarthi Memorial Medical College, Kanpur, India

The Pediatric Eye

1

Vikas Kanaujia, Rajat M. Srivastava, Isha Chaturvedi, and Priya Singh

1.1 Introduction

A pediatric eye is not merely a miniature of an adult, rather is a 'system under evolution'. It represents the complex interplay of the developing eye and the brain resulting in the gift of vision. Unlike an adult, the optical system in children is highly dynamic and any pathology affecting it can have far-reaching consequences. As clinicians, it is imperative for us to have an insight into the process of visual development and maturation to ensure optimal visual outcomes while treating children. Pediatric cataract management requires a dynamic approach. The efforts required do not end with a good cataract surgery but continue all along the journey of visual rehabilitation. The aim of this chapter is to revisit the process of ocular development and understand the differences between an adult and pediatric eye.

1.2 The Developing Eye

The earliest signs of development of the eye in a vertebrate embryo are observed as early as by the third week of gestation and this process of development and maturation of the visual system continues till about 16 years of age [1, 2]. This entire process of visual development may be classified into the following phases: ***Intra-uterine phase, phase of Postnatal Ocular growth, and phase of Emmetropization and visual maturation***. In contrast to the intra-uterine phase, the phases of ocular growth and emmetropization are intertwined and occur simultaneously (Fig. 1.1).

V. Kanaujia · I. Chaturvedi · P. Singh
Department of Ophthalmology, Sanjay Gandhi Post Graduate Institute of Medical Sciences, Lucknow, India

R. M. Srivastava (✉)
Department of Ophthalmology, King George's Medical University, Lucknow, India

S. Agrawal (ed.), *Pediatric Cataract*,
https://doi.org/10.1007/978-981-16-1736-2_1

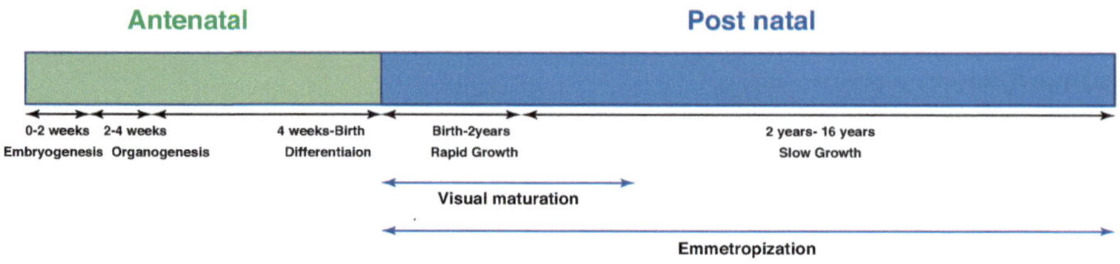

Fig. 1.1 Different phases of genesis and development of the eye

Anomalies in ocular growth during infancy and childhood can impair the process of emmetropization and can lead to suboptimal visual functions. At the same time, irregularities in the intra-uterine development can range from being embryo lethal in severe cases to congenital abnormalities in less severe instances.

The whole process of development of the embryo is meticulously orchestrated by sequential expression of genes, known as the ***Homeobox genes***. These are highly conserved regions of DNA (Deoxyribonucleic Acid) that code for proteins with specific DNA-binding capabilities. The Homeobox genes are considered as the master regulators as they regulate the expression of downstream genes involved in process of organogenesis [3]. PAX-6 gene (Paired homeoboX 6) is a specific homeobox gene identified with the development of the eye [1]. It is expressed very early in the region of head ectoderm, marking the area for development of the primordial eye field. Other Homeobox genes that play a key role in the development of the eye include PAX2, RX, and PITX2 genes [1]. Additionally, Sonic Hedgehog gene expression is important for division of eye field into two for development of the two eyes [4].

The genetic blueprint provides for expression of growth factors, ligands, and morphogens involved in the development and differentiation of ocular structures [5]. The concentration gradients of these molecules determine the fate of cells and tissues. These ligands and growth factors act either by direct interaction with the intracellular receptors or via surface receptors inducing a cascade of intracellular signalling. Such interactions are responsible for regulating gene expression affecting growth and differentiation of cells including their intracellular remodelling, protein trafficking, cell motility etc. This cascade of events is initially regulated by maternal messenger RNA (Ribonucleic Acid) till about stage of midblastula, when the embryonic genome takes over this process [1].

1.3 The Intra-uterine Phase

Our visual system is unique as the optic nerve unlike any other nerve is comparable to the white matter of the brain both of which have the same embryological origin. Similarly, the retina has been regarded as modified brain cortex, on basis of its embryonic origin [6]. The intra-uterine phase of development of the eye involves the stages of development of embryo ***(embryogenesis)***, development of the eye anlage

Table 1.1 Ocular and adnexal derivatives from different embryonic tissues

Embryonic tissue	Derivatives
Neural ectoderm	Smooth muscle of iris Optic vesicle and cup Iris epithelium Ciliary epithelium Part of vitreous Retina Retinal pigment epithelium Fibres of optic nerve
Surface ectoderm	Conjunctival epithelium Corneal epithelium Lacrimal glands Tarsal glands Lens
Mesoderm	Extra-ocular muscles Sclera Vascular endothelium of eye and orbit Choroid Part of vitreous
Neural Crest	Corneal stroma, keratocytes, endothelium Sclera Trabecular meshwork endothelium Iris stroma Ciliary muscles Choroidal stroma Part of vitreous Uveal and conjunctival melanocytes Meningeal sheaths of the optic nerve Ciliary ganglion Schwann cells of nerve sheaths Orbital bones and connective tissue Muscular layer of blood vessels

(organogenesis), and differentiation of ocular structures ***(differentiation)***. Majority of the eye and orbital structures are ***ectomesenchymal*** (neural crest cell derived) and ***neuroectodermal*** in origin with inputs from the surface ectoderm and mesoderm (Table 1.1) [1]. Since neural crest cells (NCC) also make key contributions to facial, dental, and calvarial structures, syndromes that arise from neural crest maldevelopment (e.g., Goldenhar syndrome) often involve the eye along with facial and dental abnormalities [1]. Following landmark events during the intra-uterine development of the eye may be referred to while understanding the process of development.

1.3.1 Formation of the Germ Layers

Following fertilization, the ovum undergoes a series of cell divisions progressing from 2 cells to 16 cell stages. At this stage of embryogenesis, it resembles a mulberry and is termed as ***Morula.*** The cells in Morula reorganize into inner cell mass

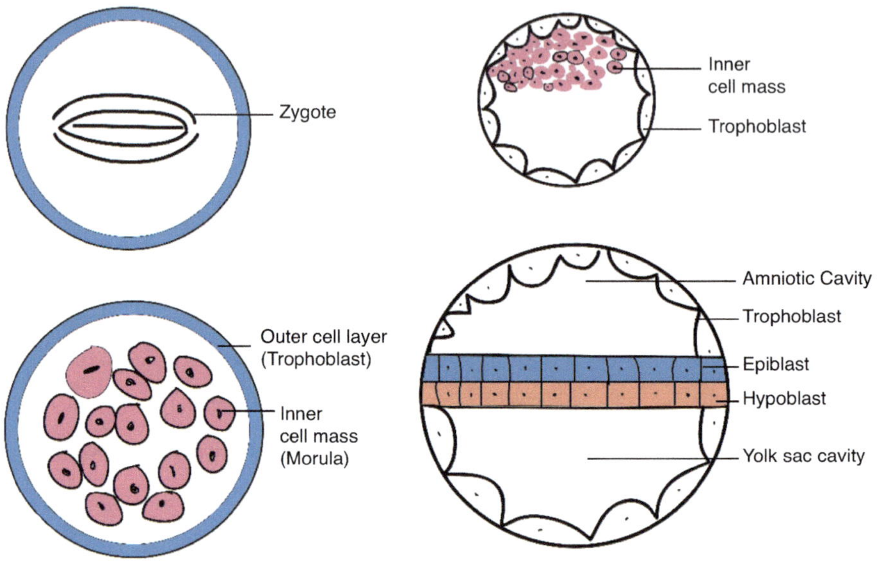

Fig. 1.2 The impregnated ovum undergoes rapid cell division to differentiate into an outer cell layer (trophoblast) and inner cell mass to form Morula (images on left). Subsequently, Blastocyst forms (top right image). The trophoblast forms the placenta and the inner cell mass forms two layers of cells, the epiblast and the hypoblast (bottom right image)

and outer cell layer. The outer cells and inner cell mass is separated by ingress of fluid and this transforms Morula into a cyst, called as the ***Blastocyst***. The outer cells in Blastocyst give rise to ***trophoblast*** whereas the inner cell mass differentiates to form the ***embryoblast***. The embryoblast is eccentrically attached to the trophoblast at one pole and separated by a fluid-filled cavity from the rest of the trophoblast (Fig. 1.2) [7].

The inner cell mass subsequently undergoes differentiation to form a layer of a columnar cells and a layer of cubical cells known as ***Epiblast*** and ***Hypoblast***, respectively. The epiblast layer eventually forms the ***Ectoderm*** (outer germinal layer) whereas hypoblast forms the ***Endoderm*** (inner germinal layer). At this stage, some of the cells of the ectoderm undergo proliferation to form an 'elevated tissue mass' known as the ***Primitive Streak***. The proliferating cells from the primitive streak invaginate and spread between the ectoderm and endoderm forming the third germinal layer, the ***Mesoderm***. Mesoderm separates the outer and inner germinal at all places except in the region of ***Prochordal Plate*** cranially and ***Cloacal Membrane*** caudally. Thus, all the three germinal layers of embryo are developed from which all the organs are formed. This process of formation and differentiation of germinal layers along with the development of primitive streak is known as ***Gastrulation*** (Fig. 1.3).

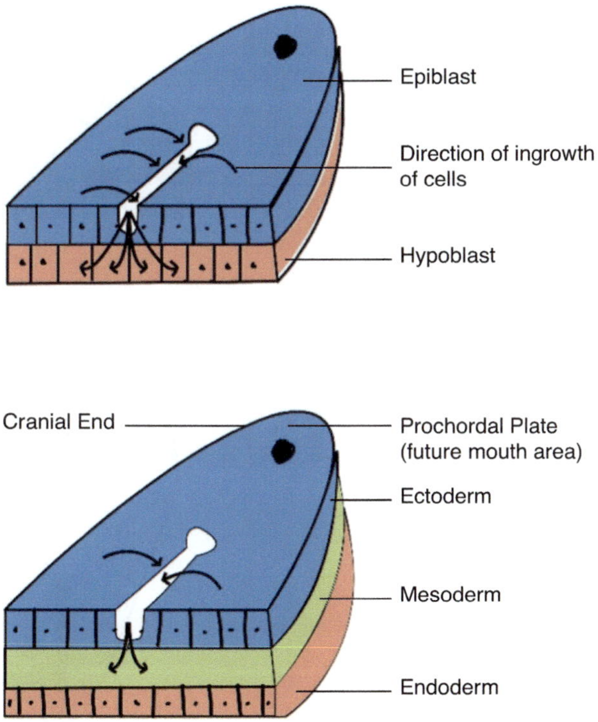

Fig. 1.3 Gastrulation and the formation of the three germ layers. Proliferating cells from the primitive streak invaginate between ectoderm and endoderm to form the mesoderm except in the regions of prochordal plate (cranially) and cloacal membrane (caudally)

1.3.2 Formation of Neural Tube

As the embryo develops, the cells from the cranial end of the primitive streak invaginate to form a cord-like structure extending up to the prochordal plate. This cord-like structure present in the midline of the embryo surrounded by the mesoderm is known as the ***Notochord***. The ectoderm overlying the region of notochord thickens to form a distinctive plate known as the ***Neural Plate*** which eventually differentiates into ***Neuroectoderm*** (Fig. 1.4). The region of mesoderm lying adjacent to the notochord is referred to as the ***Paraxial Mesoderm*** whereas the peripheral mesoderm is called ***Visceral Mesoderm***. The cells present at the edges of the neural ectoderm differentiate to form ***Neural Crest Cells*** (Fig. 1.5). These are transient migratory cells that migrate to various regions of the developing embryo to form different tissue structures.

The neural plate subsequently gets depressed in the midline to form a groove called ***Neural Groove***. As the groove gets deeper, the edges of the plate become prominent and grow closer, converting the groove into a tube-like structure known

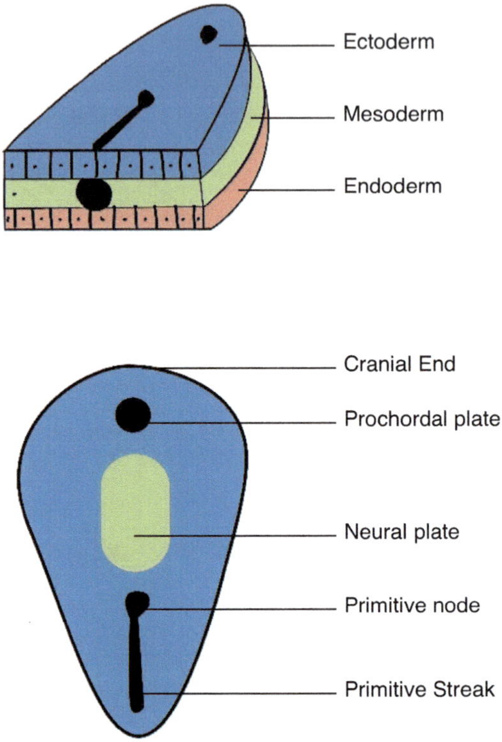

Fig. 1.4 Formation of neural plate and differentiation into neuroectoderm

as ***Neural Tube***. The closure of the groove begins centrally before proceeding cranially and caudally (Fig. 1.5). The cranial end of the tube is widened and develops into brain whereas the narrow caudal end forms the spinal cord. Eyes develop from grooves in the lateral walls of cranial end of the neural tube.

1.3.3 Formation of the Eye

As the closure of the neural groove progresses, two depressions are observed to develop in the lateral walls of the cranial end of the neural grooves known as the ***Optic Pits***. With the closure of the cranial end of the neural groove, it transforms into a closed structure called the ***Prosencephalic Vesicle,*** which eventually forms the brain. The optic pits in the lateral walls prosencephalic vesicle (cranial neural tube) deepen to form the ***Optic Sulcus*** (Fig. 1.5). The sulcus on either side enlarge and appear as rounded projection springing from the lateral aspects of the developing brain and are termed as the ***Optic Vesicles***. These optic vesicles arising as lateral outpouchings of the neural ectoderm are in direct contact with the surface ectoderm unlike the rest of neural tube, which is surrounded by a layer of paraxial mesoderm. As these grow laterally, the connection between the optic vesicle with the neural tube gets narrowed and elongated to form the ***Optic Stalk*** (Fig. 1.6). At this stage,

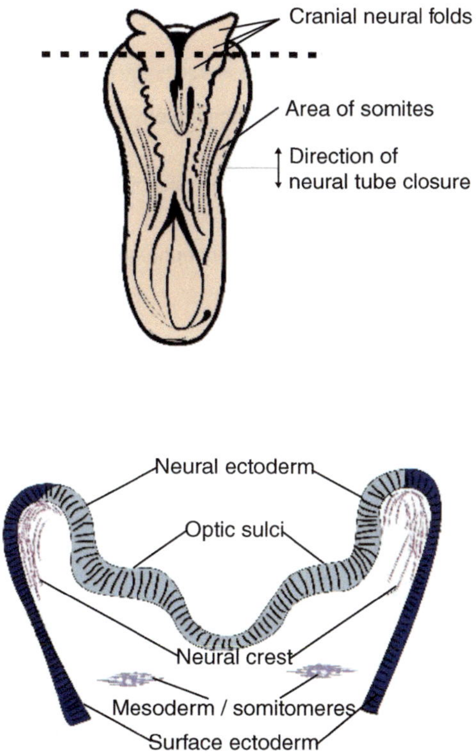

Fig. 1.5 Embryo showing closure of neural groove in central part (above) and cross-section at the dotted line (below)

optic vesicle and the stalk get surrounded by a layer of paraxial mesoderm and only the most prominent area of the optic vesicle is in direct contact with the surface ectoderm (Fig. 1.7) [8].

The region of surface ectoderm overlying the optic vesicle undergoes thickening to form the ***Lens Plate*** or the ***Lens Placode***. This is followed by sinking of the lens placode that separates from the surface ectoderm to form a hollow sphere known as the ***Lens Vesicle***. Simultaneously, growth and enlargement of the optic vesicle are observed. The lens vesicle is invaginated into the optic vesicle by asymmetric growth observed in the upper and lower portion of the optic vesicle with its margins rimming around the lens vesicle (Fig. 1.8). The optic vesicle gets folded upon itself to form a bilayered structure known as the ***Optic Cup*** with the lens vesicle occupying the central concavity of the cup. The invagination progresses rapidly until the inner wall of the optic vesicle merges with the outer wall. The inner wall of the optic cup will eventually differentiate to form the ***Neurosensory Retina*** whereas the outer wall will form the ***Retinal Pigment Epithelium*** (Fig. 1.9).

Due to asymmetrical growth of the optic vesicle during the process of invagination, a groove is formed along the ventral aspect (underside) of the developing eye extending from the cup margins anteriorly to the optic stalk posteriorly. This groove is known as the ***Choroidal Fissure*** or the ***Fetal Fissure*** (Fig. 1.9). Deficient closure of this groove results in development of ocular coloboma (Fig. 1.10) [8].

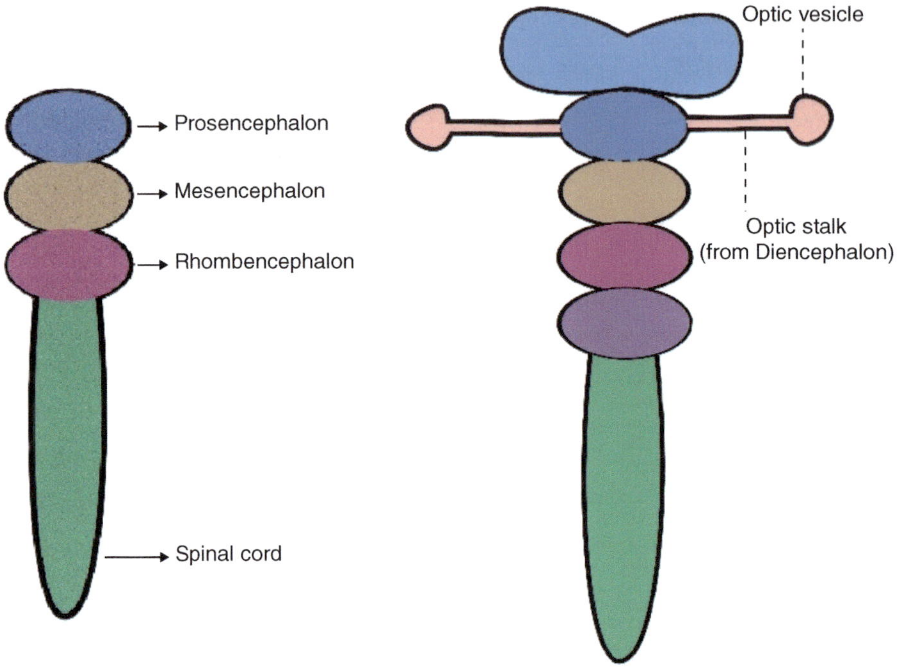

Fig. 1.6 Differentiation of neural tube and development of optic vesicle. Prosencephalon differentiates into Telencephalon and Diencephalon. Optic vesicles arrises from the Diencephalon

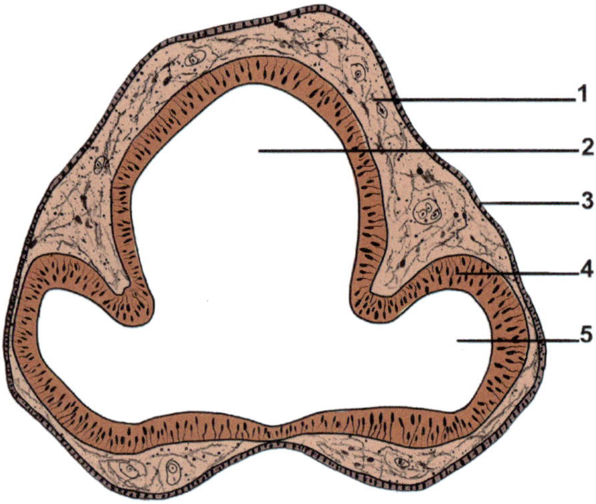

Fig. 1.7 Optic vesicle development in relation to surface ectoderm. (**1**) Mesoderm; (**2**) Cavity of forebrain; (**3**) Surface ectoderm; (**4**) Wall of optic vesicle; (**5**) Cavity of the optic vesicle. Surface ectoderm overlies very closely to the prominent portion of optic vesicle. (Modified and redrawn from Mann I. A general outline of the development of optic vesicle and the associated mesoderm. The development of the human eye. 2nd ed; 1950)

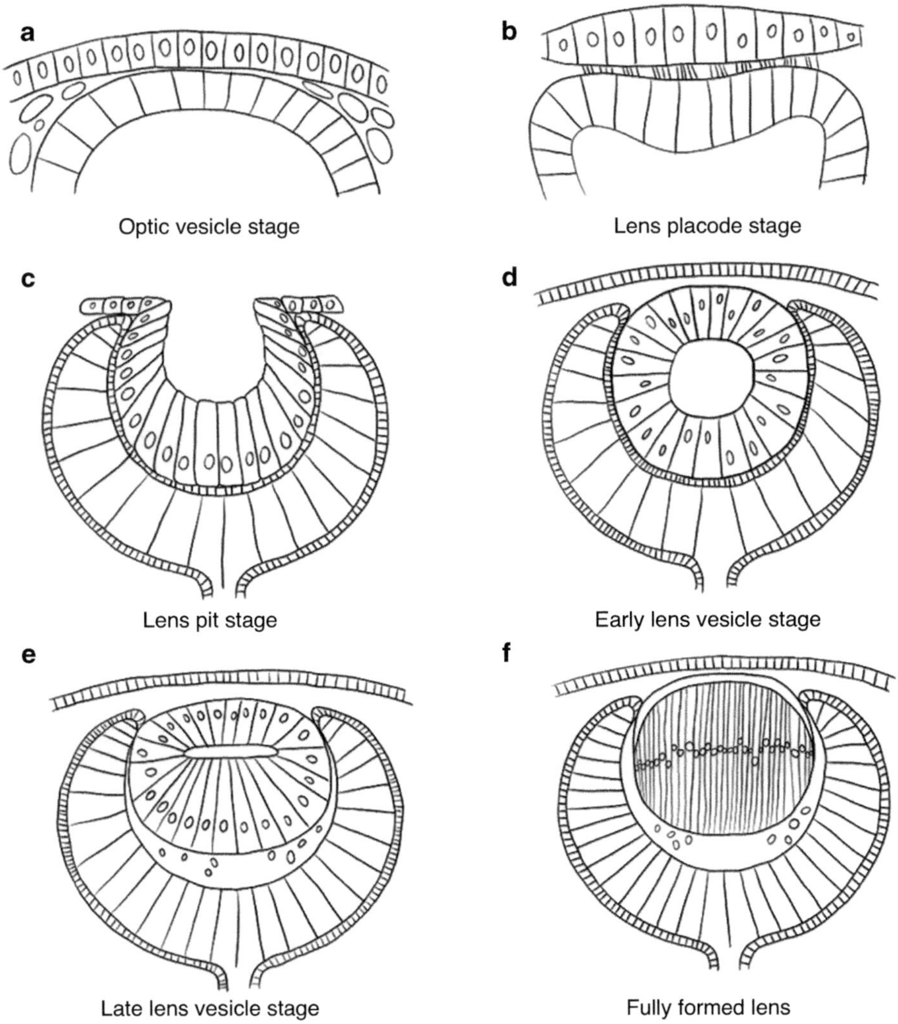

Fig. 1.8 Development and invagination of the lens vesicle. Various stages of development are highlighted in Figs. (**a**) to (**f**)

At this stage, the anterior margins of the optic cup rim around the lens vesicle and a layer of surface ectoderm overlies the structure. The groove on the underside is filled by the paraxial mesoderm, which also fills in the space between the lens vesicle and the optic cup separating them. Conglomeration of neural crest cells is found around the junction of anterior margins of the optic cup with the lens vesicle. The developing optic cup is surrounded by mesoderm. The mesoderm entering the choroidal fissure forms the initial blood vessels (***Hyaloid Artery***), which supplies

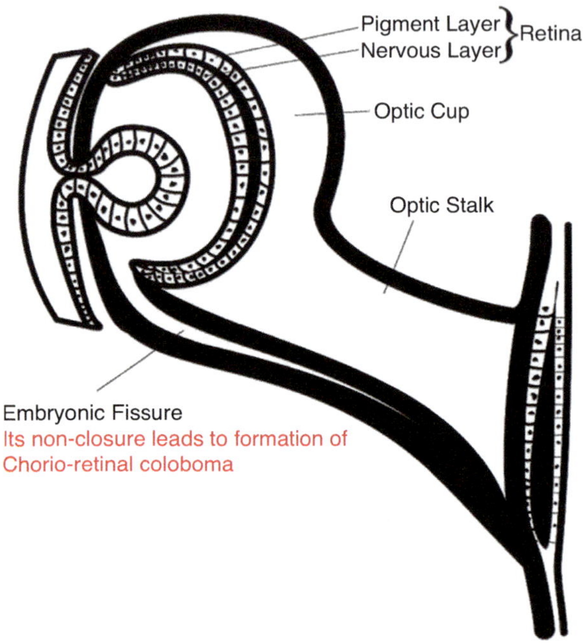

Fig. 1.9 Development of the human optic cup in 28-day embryo. The wall of the cup has been cut to demonstrate the two layers. The lens vesicle has been opened to demonstrate the cavity and narrow passage running from this through the lens stalk

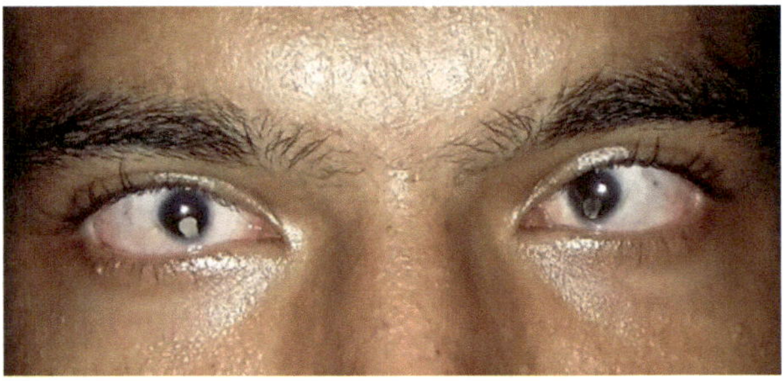

Fig. 1.10 Micropthalmos with iris coloboma and cataract

the primitive ocular structures including the developing lens (Fig. 1.11) [8]. The choroidal fissure then begins to close, beginning in the centre, proceeding anteriorly and posteriorly to complete the basic framework of the developing eye. These structures will subsequently undergo further development and differentiation to evolve into an eye of an infant. The details of further growth and differentiation of various ocular structures shall be discussed in the following section.

1.3.4 Development and Differentiation of Ocular Structures

Following the formation of the optic cup and the lens vesicle, the structures of the eye undergo further development and differentiate into their functional forms. We shall now study how various ocular structures in the primitive eye evolve into an

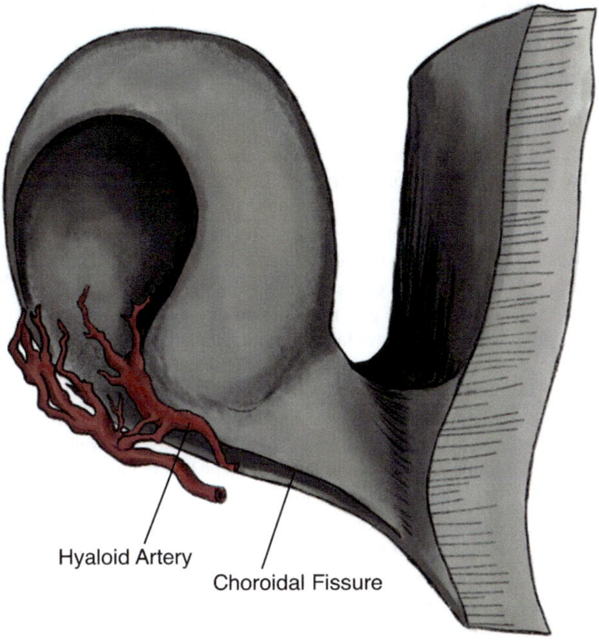

Fig. 1.11 Development of blood vessels through the Choroidal Fissure (Modified and redrawn from Mann I. A general outline of the development of optic vesicle and the associated mesoderm. The development of the human eye. 2nd ed; 1950)

eye of a full-term infant. The chronology of important events during embryological development of eye is mentioned in Table 1.2.

1.3.4.1 Cornea and Anterior Chamber

With the separation and subsequent invagination of the lens vesicle, the defect overlying the optic cup is filled by a layer of surface ectoderm. This layer of surface ectoderm forms the ***Primitive Corneal Epithelium*** [9]. This bilayered structure gives rise to ***Primary Corneal Stroma*** by gradual subepithelial addition of fibrillar elements, which would eventually condense to form the ***Bowman's layer*** [10, 11]. Primary corneal epithelium finally differentiates to form the four-layered stratified corneal epithelium along with the epithelial basement membrane to complete the process of development of the corneal epithelium. At this time, proliferation of cells from an undifferentiated conglomerate of cells lying near the anterior margins of the optic cup is seen. This undifferentiated cell mass is of neural crest cell origin. Three distinct waves of cellular proliferation from this cell mass are observed which are responsible for further development of the cornea and the anterior segment structures of the eye (Fig. 1.12) [1, 12].

The ***first wave of cells*** from this mass grow in the space between the lens vesicle and the surface ectoderm (which forms the primitive corneal epithelium). This wave results in the formation of ***Corneal Endothelium***. ***Descemet's Membrane***, which is the basement membrane of the corneal endothelial cells is subsequently laid. Initially, the surface epithelium and the corneal endothelial layer of the developing cornea lie in close approximation until the third wave of cells comes to lie between them.

Table 1.2 Important chronological events of ocular development

Embryo age	Event	Associated anomaly
22 days	Appearance of optic pits.	
25 days	Optic pits accentuate optic vesicles attached to diencephalon by optic stalk. Neural crest cells migrate to surround the optic vesicles.	Primary anophthalmia occurs due to failure of elongation of optic pits to form optic vesicles.
28 days	Formation of lens placodes by thickening of surface ectoderm on top of optic vesicle.	
33 days	Lens vesicle gets separated from the surface ectoderm. Optic vesicle gets transformed into a double-walled optic cup. Outer layer of optic cup later evolves as retinal pigment epithelium (RPE) and inner as neurosensory retina.	Failure of lens vesicle separation causes Type II Peters Anomaly with keratolenticular adhesions.
	Ventral part of the optic cup has a deficiency known as choroidal or embryonic fissure To complete the wall of the globe, the two lips of the embryonic fissure meet and fuse.	Failure of fusion of embryonic fissure lips results in the formation of typical colobomas.
35 days	Hyaloid artery enters optic cup via optic fissure, primary lens fibres start forming (embryonic nucleus), migration of neural crest wave.	
6–8 weeks	Appearance of eyelid folds, migration of retinal cells begins, neural crest cells of corneal endothelium and stroma migrate, cavity of lens vesicle obliterates, secondary vitreous surrounds hyaloid system, choroidal vasculature develops.	
9–12 weeks	Secondary lens fibres (fetal nucleus) laid down by equatorial cells of anterior epithelium of lens vesicle. Precursors of rods and cones differentiate. Anterior rim of optic vesicle grows forward. Ciliary body starts to develop. Fusion of eyelid folds occurs.	Defective maturation of secondary lens fibres leads to microspherophakia.
13–16 weeks	Initiation of regression of hyaloid artery and development of retinal vessels starts. Iris sphincter, Descemet membrane and Schlemm canal form.	
17–20 weeks	Development of photoreceptors, differentiation of choroid, vascularization of iris stroma and initiation of separation of eyelids occurs.	
21–28 weeks	Differentiation of retinal layers, formation of dilator muscles of iris and ciliary muscle in ciliary body occurs.	
29–32 weeks	Completion of regression of hyaloid system and formation of anterior chamber angle.	Failure of regression of hyaloid system causes persistent fetal vasculature (PFV).
32–36 weeks	Completion of optic nerve fibres myelination, retinal vascularization up to periphery and disappearance of pupillary membrane.	

A ***second wave of cells*** from the neural crest cells is observed to grow between the corneal endothelium and the lens vesicle. This layer results in the formation of the ***Iris Stroma and muscles***. Cells from mesodermal origin also are observed to infiltrate resulting in formation of the blood vessels. The anterior continuation of the pigmented layer of the optic cup gives rise to the ***pigmented epithelium***

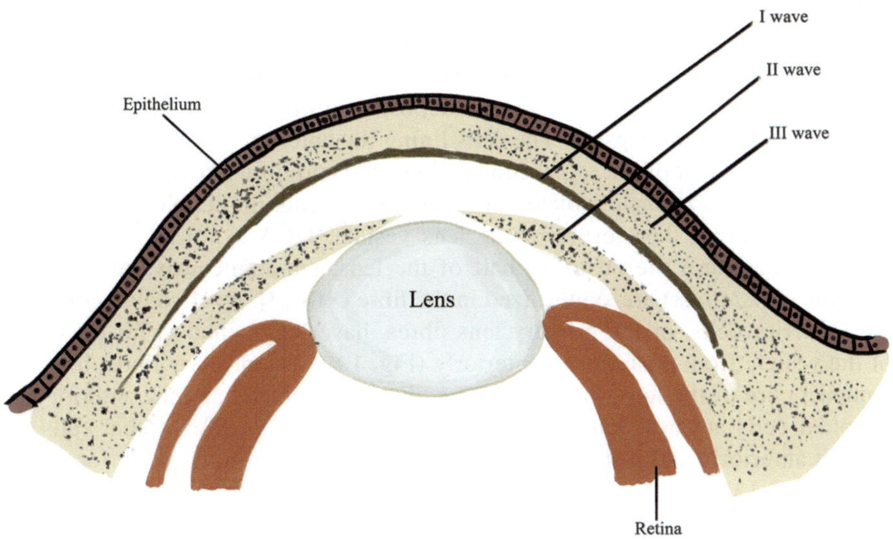

Fig. 1.12 Migration and in the growth of neural crest cells and formation of anterior chamber structures. I: First wave forms corneal endothelium; II: Second wave forms iris stroma; III: Third wave forms corneal stroma (keratocytes) (Modified and redrawn from Bron A.J, Tripathi R, Tripathi B.J. Development of the human eye. Wolff's anatomy of the eye and orbit. 8th ed; 1997)

of the Iris and the Ciliary body. At this stage, cells from mesodermal origin lie between the corneal endothelium and lens practically leaving no space between them. Subsequently, multiple small vacuoles are seen to develop between corneal endothelium and lens. These vacuoles join to form an anatomically empty space resulting in formation of the ***rudimentary anterior chamber***. With the development of iris tissue by this second wave, the cavity is divided into anterior and posterior chambers [13]. The physiological anterior and posterior chamber containing circulating aqueous humour is formed only after the development of ciliary body and the angle of the eye [8].

A ***third wave of cells*** from the mass of neural crest cells is seen to insinuate between the corneal epithelium and the endothelial layers. This wave of mesenchymal cells results in formation of the ***Secondary Corneal Stroma***. Primary corneal stroma acts like a scaffold for the invading keratocytes for lamellar and regular arrangement of collagen fibrils. This arrangement of collagen fibrils is seen in the central and posterior stroma. Anterior stroma continues to consist of the condensed acellular fibrils forming the Bowman's membrane. By third month of gestation, corneal nerves invade the stroma and eventually penetrate the Bowman's layer to enter corneal epithelium. Simultaneously, the density of functioning Na^+/K^+ ATPase metabolic pump over the endothelium increases, which makes the cornea transparent in utero [14, 15]. Thus, the cornea of a full-term newborn almost closely resembles to that of an adult barring some differences which are neutralized by further development in the postnatal period.

1.3.4.2 Crystalline Lens

The crystalline lens is purely derived from the surface ectoderm. The lens vesicle at this stage contains a single layer of cuboidal cells surrounding a large lumen. The epithelial cells of the lens vesicle deposit additional basal lamina material, which forms the lens capsule. The cells lining the anterior capsule remain cuboidal whereas the rest of the cells become elongated and fibre like filling up the lens vesicle. The lens capsule isolates the lens constituents immunologically within the globe. During the closure of the lens vesicle, DNA synthesis decreases in the cells that form the posterior half of the lens; simultaneously, specific lens proteins (*crystallins*) are synthesized in the fibre cells [3]. By 45 days' gestation, the posterior cells, or the primary lens fibres, have lengthened to fill the cavity of the vesicle from posterior to anteriorly (Fig. 1.8). The primary fibres form the compact core of the lens, known as the ***embryonic nucleus*** and the anterior lens cuboidal cells are now known as lens epithelial cells. Lens epithelial cells are present anteriorly and just posterior to the equator but not in the posterior part of lens (Fig. 1.13).

The pre-equatorial epithelial cells retain their mitotic activity throughout life, producing the secondary lens fibres (*fetal nucleus*). These fibres are displaced inward between the capsule and the embryonic nucleus and meet on the vertical planes, the lens sutures. The first suture marking the fetal nucleus is shaped like a Y anteriorly and an inverted Y posteriorly. At first, the lens is spherical, but it becomes ellipsoid with the addition of secondary fibres [12]. In the third month, the innermost fibres mature; cytoplasmic fibrillar material increases and cellular organelles decrease. The equatorial diameter of the unfixed human lens measures 2 mm at 12 weeks and 6 mm at 35 weeks. Both the growth and the maturation of lenticular fibres continue throughout life.

During fetal development, nucleus of the lens is enveloped within a nutritive support structure supplied by the hyaloid artery known as tunica vasculosa lentis, which regresses by birth (Fig. 1.16) [8]. The zonular apparatus forms mainly from ectomesenchymal cells as a part of vitreous and ciliary body.

1.3.4.3 Uvea and Sclera

The iris and the ciliary body develop from the anterior extension of bilayered neuroectoderm of the optic cup [12]. The stroma of ciliary body and the choroid are formed by extensions from the mass of neural crest cells. A layer of paraxial mesoderm around the optic cup condenses to form the muscles and blood supply of the uveal tract. Also, the mesoderm condenses near the margins of the optic cup to form the cores of the ciliary processes lined by the pigmented and non-pigmented epithelium of the optic cup. The choroidal net seems to develop wherever the mesoderm is in contact with the outer pigmented layer of the optic cup. Thus, it is found deficient in regions where the choroidal fissure has not closed (coloboma) or lacks pigmented epithelium [8].

The sclera is predominantly neural crest cell derived except for a small temporal portion, which is mesodermal in origin [16]. Its development proceeds from anterior to posterior, from the fibrous condensation of mesenchyme originating from the neural crest cells anteriorly to the optic nerve posteriorly. The sclera joins the

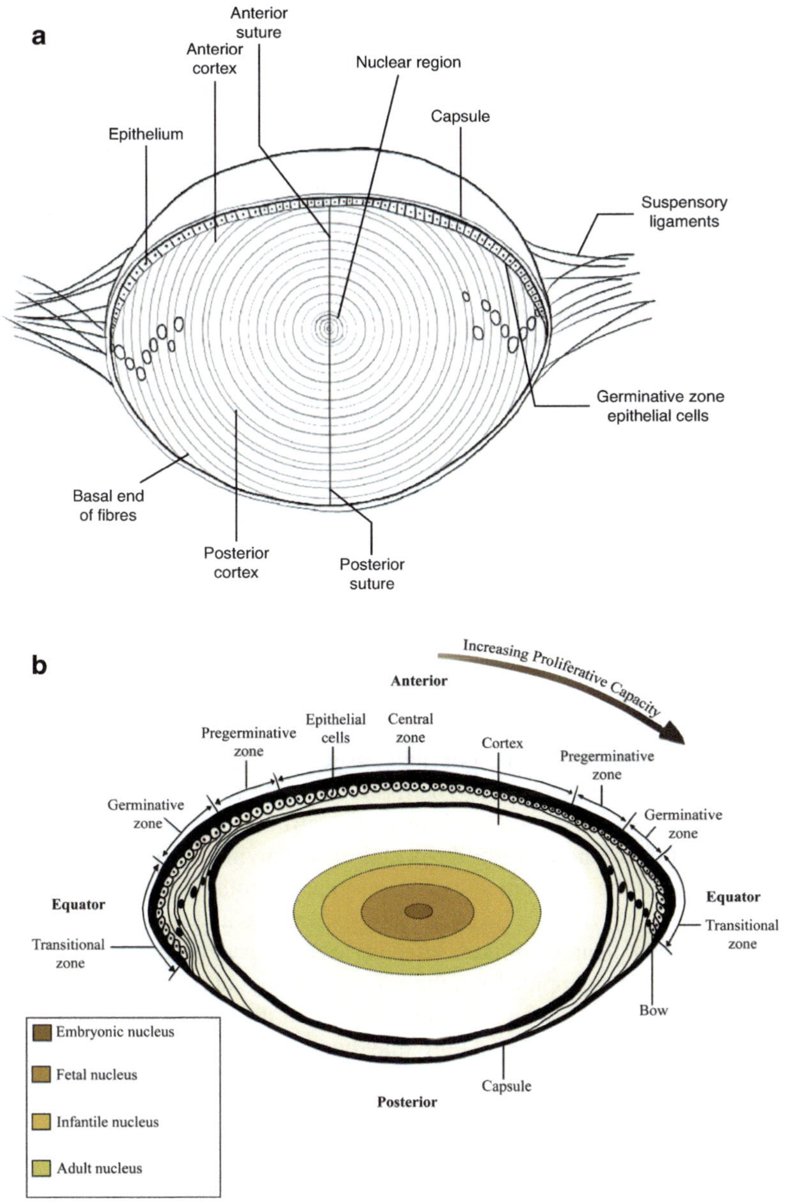

Fig. 1.13 (**a**) Formation of lens fibres and sutures (**b**) Crystalline lens in an adult

developing cornea near the equator of the eye before it expands to surround the developing optic cup. The anterior sclera is fully formed by 7 weeks of gestation followed by equatorial and posterior sclera [17]. Alike choroid, its development too seems to be dependent upon contact with pigmented epithelium of the retina. The sclera is mainly composed of fibroblast, collagen and proteoglycans.

1.3.4.4 Trabecular Meshwork

The primordium of the trabecular meshwork is formed by mass of undifferentiated cells from neural crest cell origin lying near the anterior edge of the developing optic cup [18, 19]. The same mass of tissue also gives rise to the corneal endothelium and stroma, iris and ciliary body. The mesenchymal cells destined to form the trabecular meshwork lie loosely attached with each other. These cells differentiate to form collagen fibrils and elastic tissue which evolve into trabecular beams. The cells also produce glycosaminoglycans and glycoproteins, which constitute the extracellular matrix of trabecular beams. The entire cell mass is initially covered by the corneal endothelium with iris inserted onto the endothelium. With time, there is posterior migration of the uveal tissue, which uncovers the trabecular meshwork [20]. The outer part of the trabecular meshwork forms a part of corneal stroma and is known as the ***corneo-scleral trabecular meshwork*** and the inner part covered by uveal tissue forms the ***uveal meshwork*** [12]. It is postulated that with further development, the endothelium covering the trabecular meshwork undergoes excavation and atrophy with enlargement of the trabecular meshwork spaces. With deepening of the recess of the angle of the eye, direct communication is established between the trabecular meshwork and the anterior chamber. Any deficiency in the process of differentiation of the primordial trabecular meshwork cells lead to ***trabeculo-dysgenesis*** leading to development of congenital glaucoma.

1.3.4.5 Retina and Vitreous

Following the formation of the bilayered optic cup, the space between the lens vesicle and the cup is filled by mesodermal tissue. This mesoderm enters the cavity of the cup via the choroidal fissure. The tissue differentiates to form vascular channel supplying nutrition to the developing ocular structures including lens. Thus, the vascular component along with fibrils and mesenchymal tissue constitute ***Primary Vitreous*** [12]. As the development proceeds, the vascular structures undergo degeneration and primary vitreous is replaced by hyalocytes and type II collagen fibrils to form the optically clear ***Secondary Vitreous***. Secondary vitreous is neuroectodermal in origin with possible inputs from the ectomesenchymal tissue [21]. ***Cloquet Canal*** is a remnant of the regressed vascular system and the primary vitreous (Fig. 1.14). The remnants of the fetal vasculature may be observed clinically at the optic nerve head (***Bergmeister Papilla***) and posterior pole of lens (***Mittendorf Dot***) [22].

The optic cup may be divided into two parts—anterior 1/5th called ***Pars Ciliaris Retinae*** and posterior 4/5th known as ***Pars Optica Retinae*** [23]. The former is involved in the development of the iris and ciliary body and the later in responsible for the development of retina proper. As already mentioned before, the inner layer of the optic forms the neurosensory retina whereas the outer layer forms the pigmented layer of retina. A potential space is present between these layers and is responsible for causing retinal detachment, which is actually the separation of neurosensory retina from the retinal pigment epithelium.

The differentiation and maturation of retinal tissues proceeds concentrically, beginning around the centre of the macula and extending peripherally. In the initial phase of development, there is thickening of the inner neurosensory layer of the

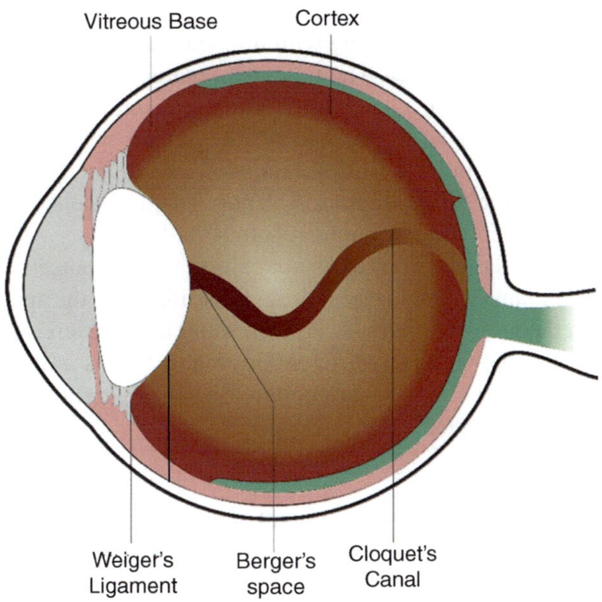

Fig. 1.14 Cloquet canal in adult vitreous

optic cup. The inner layer differentiates into three distinctive regions; the innermost ***Marginal layer***, ***inner Neuroblastic*** and ***outer Neuroblastic layers*** [22]. The marginal layer is free of any nucleated cells and mainly consists of the axons of the cells forming the ***nerve fibre layer***. The cells of inner neuroblastic layer differentiate to form the ***Ganglion cells***, ***Amacrine cells*** and the ***Muller cells***. Ganglion cells are the first to differentiate in neurosensory retina followed by the ***Bipolar and Horizontal Cells***, which develop from the cells in the outer neuroblastic layer. The last of the cells to differentiate are the ***Photoreceptors (Cones and Rods)*** derived from the outer neuroblastic layer [12]. A cell-free zone formed by tangled cell processes between the inner and outer neuroblastic layer known as the ***transient layer of Chievtz*** differentiates to form the ***inner plexiform layer*** whereas the axonal connections between the bipolar cells and the photoreceptors give rise to the ***outer plexiform layer*** [12]. The adjacent lateral surfaces of the photoreceptors join to form the ***external limiting membrane***. The cell membrane of photoreceptor and retinal pigment epithelium form junctional complexes, obliterating the space between the neurosensory and pigment epithelium layers.

The structural reorganization of macula and fovea continues throughout intrauterine phase and reach maturity by 3–4 years of age. By the 22nd gestational week, most of the layers of neurosensory retina are formed in the region of macula with consistent increase in cone density in the foveal region. A depression in the region corresponding with fovea is observed around 24th to 26th week with thinning of the ganglion and inner nuclear layers. The bases of photoreceptors are tapered and displaced laterally to form the Henle's layer. This makes the foveal dip more prominent with presence of only cones. By seventh month, only acellular fibrous zone corresponding to the layer of Chievtz along with thinned out ganglion and inner nuclear layer form the slopes of the fovea. The functional maturity of the retina begins with the development of fixation in a newborn. Further structural and functional changes occurring in retina would be referred to in the section elaborating the postnatal development phase. The process of differentiation of cells in retina proceeds from the innermost cell layer to the outermost. Thus, ganglion cells and retinal nerve fibres are first to differentiate and photoreceptors the last [22].

The outer layer of the optic cup does not exhibit many changes during development. The layer remains single layered throughout life. With the appearance of pigment granules in the protoplasm of its cells, the outer layer differentiates to form the Retinal Pigment Epithelium. This differentiation also begins at the posterior pole. The retinal pigment epithelial cells are bound together by tight junctions and form the outer blood-ocular barrier.

1.3.4.6 Optic Nerve

The optic nerve develops from the optic stalk, the original connection between the optic vesicle and the forebrain. Initially, the optic stalk consists of the cells from neural ectoderm surrounded by neural crest cells. Later, these cells undergo vacuolation and degenerate making way for the axons of ganglion cells. The axons of the ganglion cells converge at the optic stalk to form the optic nerve. Migration and differentiation of the neural crest cells form the pia, arachnoid and dura mater of the optic nerve. Myelination starts in the chiasm at the seventh month of gestation, proceeds towards the eye, and ceases at the lamina cribrosa by about 1 month after birth (Fig. 1.15). The optic nerve is believed to be analogous to the white matter of the brain.

1.3.4.7 Intra-ocular Blood Supply

All the vascular supply of the eye is mesodermal and neuroectodermal in origin. The paraxial mesoderm around the optic vesicle differentiates to form the endothelium whereas the neuroectoderm contributes to the connective tissue sheath and muscular layer of blood vessels. These blood vessels gain entry into the eye through the choroidal fissure. The vessels in the choroidal fissure form two sets of freely anastomosing vessels; one forming an annular ring around the margins of the optic cup and the other entering the optic cup through the fissure. The vessel entering the fissure forms the future ***Hyaloid Artery system***. It enters the eye and forms the ***fetal intra-ocular blood system***. It forms the ***Tunica Vasculosa Lentis*** supplying the crystalline lens and multiple other branches supplying the vitreous and surrounding tissues called ***Vasa Hyaloidea Propria*** (Fig. 1.16) [8].

Most of the fetal intra-ocular blood system atrophies and is replaced by secondary vitreous. The definitive blood supply of retina is formed at a later stage. The retinal blood vessels follow the same pattern of differentiation as the retina, beginning from the centre and spreading concentrically to the periphery. The vascularization of the peripheral retina is completed by 40 weeks of gestation. Persistence of intra-ocular fetal vasculature can result in congenital cataract with Persistent

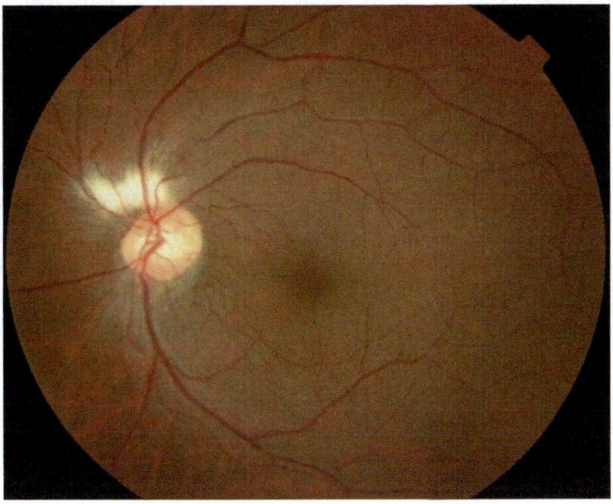

Fig. 1.15 Myelinated nerve fibres are visible when the myelination exceeds beyond the lamina cribrosa. Their clinical relevance is limited to an enlarged blind spot on perimetry

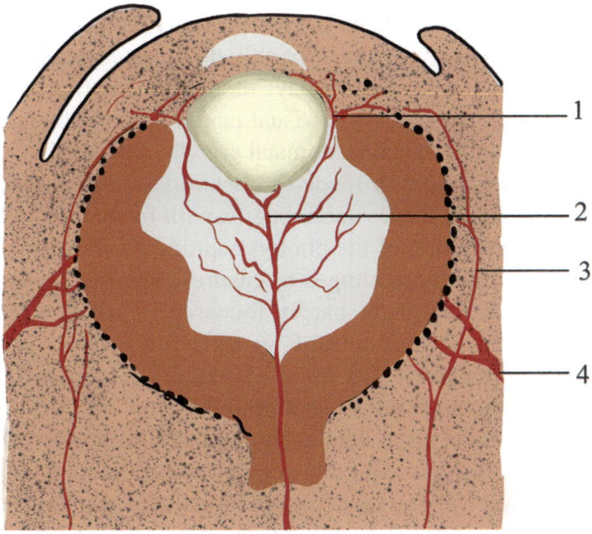

1. Annular vessel; 3. Choroidal vessel;
2. Hyaloid artery; 4. Vortex vein.

Fig. 1.16 Fetal intra-ocular blood system (Hyaloid Artery) (Modified and redrawn from Mann I. A general outline of the development of optic vesicle and the associated mesoderm. The development of the human eye. 2nd ed; 1950)

Hyperplastic Primary Vitreous (PHPV) now termed as Persistent Fetal Vasculature (PFV). Similarly, premature babies may have inadequate retinal vascularization causing Retinopathy of Prematurity (ROP). The paraxial mesoderm also forms the blood vessels comprising the extra-ocular blood system supplying the extra-ocular muscles, orbit, lids and adnexa.

The neural crest cells along with paraxial and maxillary mesoderm surrounding the eye differentiate to form the extra-ocular muscles, lids, conjunctiva and orbit.

The developing optic vesicle provides stimulus to the surrounding mesoderm and ectomesenchymal tissues to not only form the extra-ocular muscles but also facial structures. The lids during development are initially fused and later get separated by about 26 weeks of gestation. The optical axes of the eyes along with other ocular structures continue to change all throughout the intra-uterine phase and continue to change even in the postnatal period. By birth, the ocular structures have already undergone a tremendous amount of remodelling in utero to be functionally prepared for providing vision. However, there still remains a journey for an infant eye before it evolves into a masterpiece of an adult visual system. We shall now study how the visual system of a full-term infant evolves through the phases of postnatal ocular growth and emmetropization into an adult eye.

1.4 The Phases of Postnatal Growth, Emmetropization and Visual Maturation

Vision is an outcome of a complex neuro-physiological process involving the eye and the brain. The eye here acts as a camera providing a sharply focussed image for the brain to perceive and interpret. The visual system in an infant at birth though is formed, is still immature. Not only do the eyes and brain change anatomically with the growth of an infant, the physiological interaction between them evolves overtime to complete the process of visual maturation. Following the intra-uterine phase, the processes of postnatal anatomical growth and visual maturation occur together.

Visual maturation involves consolidation of the neural connections between the brain and the eyes and it begins with formation of image upon the retina leading to stimulation of the photoreceptors. As the eyes grow, the optical system of the eye undergoes changes to ensure a sharply focussed image upon the retina. This is essential as a sharply focussed image is a required stimulus for differentiation and maturation of visual pathway and visual cortex. Defocusing can affect the image quality upon retina, which then will affect the process of visual maturation and result in suboptimal vision. At the same time, binocular interaction is also required for development of ***binocular single vision***. Any deviation in growth or interaction between eyes during this phase of development could be indicative of underlying disease. We shall now study the various anatomical and physiological changes that occur in the eyes and brain during this phase before the visual system fine-tunes to provide the best quality vision (Table 1.3).

1.4.1 Ocular Dimensions

With the growth of the infant, eyes also grow. However, in comparison to body which increases 21 times, ocular growth is usually limited to only 1.8 times since birth [8]. This growth of the eyeball is essential for proper development of the facial features [24]. Increasing ocular dimensions provide the stimulus for orbit to grow which is necessary for development and growth of other facial bones. Small (microphthalmia) or absent (anophthalmia) eyeballs can adversely affect facial

Table 1.3 Differences between an infant eye and an adult eye

Characteristics	Infant eye (birth)	Adult eye (18 years)
Specular count	6000/mm^2	2400–3000/mm^2
Lens power	45 Dioptres	20 Dioptres
Anterior chamber depth	2.3–2.7 mm	3–3.5 mm
Dilator pupillae muscle	Poorly developed	Well developed
Trabecular meshwork	Covered with uveal tissue	Uncovered and freely communicating with anterior chamber
Retina	Underdeveloped. Cone density at fovea 18/100 micrometre	Well differentiated with foveal cone density 42/100 micrometre
Visual acuity	20/400–20/600	20/20
Stereopsis	Not developed	100 seconds of arc

Table 1.4 Change in dimensions of the eye (HCD = horizontal corneal diameter, K = Keratomery)

Dimensions at birth	
Axial length	14.5–15.5 mm
HCD	9.5–10.5 mm
K value	52.0 D
Increase in axial length	
0–6 months	4 mm
6 months to 1 year	2 mm
1–2 years	2 mm
2–5 years	1 mm
5–13 years	1 mm
Increase in HCD	
0–12 months	1 mm
Decrease in Keratometry	
0–6 months	6 D
6–12months	2–4 D
Adult dimensions	
Axial length	23.0–24.0 mm
HCD	12.0 mm
K value	42.0–44.0 D

growth and can lead to facial asymmetry. Maximal growth of the eye occurs in the first year. The changes in axial length, horizontal corneal diameter and keratometry are listed in Table 1.4 [2, 25].

1.4.2 Orbit

Almost all orbital bones are formed during the third month of gestation, and their ossification continues over the next several months. The eye reaches adult size by about age 3 years, but the adult dimensions of the orbit (a volume of 30 mL, a lid skin to orbital apex depth of 5 cm, and an overall quadrangular pear shape) sometimes may not be attained till 16 years. As the midface develops in puberty, the vertical dimensions of the orbit increase, achieving an adult configuration.

It must be noted that the angle between the orbital axes reduces with time. From being laterally placed in utero, the eyes are frontally placed at birth. This angle reaches about 68° at about 3 years of age (adult like) [12]. Frontal positioning of eyes is important as this allows for overlap between the visual field of each eye and thus is instrumental in developing binocular single vision and stereopsis. This displacement of orbit is thought to occur secondary to increased brain size or the wider skull base in higher mammals [8].

The orbit does not reach its normal volume when the globe is microphthalmic or anophthalmic. In these patients implants, conformers and soft tissue expanders may be used to promote orbital enlargement [26].

1.4.3 Extra-Ocular Muscles and Movements

The rectus muscles of infants are smaller, their tendons thinner and insertions about 2 mm closer to limbus than in adults [2]. With increasing growth of the sclera, the muscle insertions are displaced posteriorly to their normal sites. Conjugate horizontal movements are present at birth but vertical gaze movements fully develop by 6 months of age. Accommodation reflex and fusional convergence movements can be appreciated by 3 months. Intermittent strabismus may be frequently seen till about 3 months of age [2].

1.4.4 Cornea

The fetal cornea resembles adult cornea, by seventh month of gestation, other than size. Mild clouding of the cornea is common in premature infants and is also seen sometimes in healthy term newborns. It gradually resolves with a decrease in average corneal thickness from 691 μm at 30–32 weeks of gestation to about 564 μm at term [2]. In full-term infant the average horizontal corneal diameter is 9.8 mm, surface area is around 102 mm^2 and power is about 51 D [27, 28]. It reaches the adult size at about 2 years having horizontal diameter 11.7 mm, surface area 138 mm^2, the anterior curvature of 44.0 D and the mean corneal thickness of 540 μm [29]. These changes happen rapidly in the first 6 months after birth. The cell density of corneal endothelium is around 6000/mm^2 at birth. The cell count falls by 26% in the first year and a further 26% is lost over the next 11 years.

1.4.5 Sclera

The sclera is nearly spherical, dense connective tissue, relatively avascular, rigid and opaque. Its controlled growth, both during embryogenesis and later plays a critical role in determining the absolute size of the eye and the final refractive outcome. The sclera is comparatively thin and highly distensible at birth and losses its distensibility by 3 years of age [16]. Consequently, buphthalmos is typically observed if the rise in IOP occurs before 3 years of age. During its growth, the anterior sclera matures earlier (adult size by 2 years) compared to equatorial (adult size by 13 years) and posterior sclera (adult size by 16 years) and becomes more rigid with advancing age [30]. Pediatric sclera is one-fourth as stiff as it in adults hence even tiny incisions need to be sutured [31].

1.4.6 Iris and Pupil

Changes in iris colour occur over the first year of life with accumulation of iris pigments in iris stroma and in melanocytes. Increased immune response of the uveal tissue in children makes their eyes more prone to inflammation than adults, even after an uneventful cataract surgery [32].

The infant's pupil is physiologically smaller and often resistant to mydriasis in abnormalities associated with congenital cataract (e.g. in maternal rubella). Unlike the constrictor pupillae muscle which is well-formed by seventh month of gestation, dilator pupillae muscle begins to develop at 6 months of gestation and continues to develop several months postnatally [3, 12]. A pupil outside the range of 1.8 mm to 5.4 mm in diameter suggests an abnormality. A small pupil may require prolonged use of atropine preoperatively and extra manipulation including the use of iris retractors during surgery.

The pupillary light reflex develops by 32 weeks of gestation.

1.4.7 Anterior Chamber

Depth of anterior chamber in newborns ranges from 2.3 to 2.7 mm, which is shallower as compared to adults making intraoperative manipulations difficult. Iris insertion is near the level of scleral spur at birth and the formation of angle recess occurs during the first year with posterior migration of lens and ciliary body [33]. The cavity of anterior chamber is initially lined by flat cells, which undergo regression during development. Persistence of this layer of cells over iris results in persistent pupillary membrane.

The angle of the eye is not completely formed at birth. The anterior surface of iris which was inserted at the edge of corneal endothelium at 5 months of gestation is now inserted at the level of scleral spur along with the ciliary body at birth. The posterior migration of these structures continues for about the first year of life before the angle structures are completely formed. Initially, the trabecular meshwork is lightly pigmented and the pigmentation continues with age to give the typical appearance on gonioscopy in adults.

1.4.8 Intra-ocular Pressure

Intra-ocular pressure is lower in infants than adults and the range of normal readings varies depending on the tool used for measurement. A consistent reading of greater than 21 mm Hg should be considered suspicious [2].

1.4.9 Crystalline Lens

The crystalline lens continues to grow and change throughout life. The details are as followed:

- **Dimensions**

The equatorial diameter of the neonatal lens is about 6.5 mm at birth and its sagittal width ranges from 3.5 to 4.0 mm [12]. The diameter increases by the addition of secondary fibres to 9–10 mm in the second decade [2]. The size of the capsular bag changes from 7 mm at birth to 9.0 mm at about 2 years [34]. Due to the spheroidal structure of the neonatal lens, its anterior surface area also increases by about 80% from birth to young adulthood. The germinative zone of lens which gives rise to new lens fibres, constitutes about 10% of the surface area of lens at all times.

- **Structure**

The lens is enclosed in an elastic basement membrane known as the lens *capsule*. The capsule is thicker anteriorly where the epithelial cells secrete capsular material throughout life. The epithelial cells though present on the entire surface, have a mitotically active germinative zone as a ring anterior to lens equator. The dividing cells migrate towards the equator to start differentiating into lens fibres. Posteriorly the capsule is thinner; there is no epithelium with limited capsular material secreting ability.

The lens fibres are formed from epithelial cells described above. As they elongate, initially the cell nuclei a bow zone at equator. The fibres subsequently enlarge and differentiate with loss of cell nuclei along with other cellular organelles. The enlargement occurs due to expression of two proteins namely crystallins and major intrinsic protein. The lens sutures are formed as fully elongated fibres from opposite ends meet.

The mass of the lens consists of the *cortex* (outer fibres laid from young adulthood) and the *internal nucleus* (cells from embryogenesis to adolescence). Based on the time when these fibres were laid the internal nucleus is often divided into (from within outwards) embryonic (primary fibres), fetal (till birth), infantile or juvenile (early childhood to puberty) and adult (after puberty) nuclei [35]. By identifying the cataractous region of the lens in children it is possible to estimate the time of insult. As the cells of the lens are not sloughed but get progressively pushed towards the centre, unlike any other tissue in body, the lens fibres that differentiated at about 40 days of embryonic age, remain present in the adult nucleus. So, the oldest cells in the human body are the embryonic nucleus fibres (Fig. 1.13b).

As discussed, process of differentiation of lens fibres organizes the fibre membrane, its cytoplasm along with elimination of nuclei and organelles to minimize light scatter. The concentric shells of the fibres organize into transparent refractile optical elements. The larger protein molecules (Crystallins) repel each other preventing aggregation. Regular shape and volume of cells with minimal extracellular space and scatter elements maintain lens transparency. If a pathological process causes clumping of proteins, transparency of the lens is lost resulting in cataract formation. Nutrients and waste products diffuse through the lens capsule and are transferred by active transport through the anterior epithelium.

- **Accommodative Power**

The lens capsule ensures elasticity allowing accommodation. The changes in accommodative power of crystalline lens have been covered under emmetropization.

1.4.10 Retina

Retina evolves as a duplex structure capable of both scotopic and photopic vision with fovea providing the acuity for detailed observation [8]. The development and maturation of retina continue concentrically beginning from around the centre of macula. Formation of image over macula triggers further anatomic changes resulting in the formation of the foveal depression along with maturation of layers of retina. The development of macula continues during the initial 4 years of life and is characterized by loss of transient layer of Chievitz, macular pigmentation, formation of foveal light reflex, differentiation and increased density of cone photoreceptors in foveal region and narrowing of rod free zone [2]. These changes are responsible for improvement of visual acuity, colour and contrast functions during the postnatal period. The retinal vascularity improves and peripheral retinal vascularization is completed at the temporal ora serrata by 40 weeks of gestational age.

1.5 Visual Functions

With maturation of retinal layers and foveal differentiation, the visual functions improve with age in newborn. Various studies have shown that many aspects of visual performances, e.g. visual acuity, contrast, colour and binocularity vision are diminished in early infancy, relative to adults [36].

1.5.1 Visual Acuity

An estimate of the infant's visual acuity and its improvement with age varies depending on the methods used for measurements. The acuity estimate at birth ranges from 20/400 to 20/600 and the age of achieving adult acuity of 20/20 from 6–7 months to 3–5 years [2, 37]. Multiple factors including hypermetropia, astigmatism, suboptimal transmission and processing of visual information contribute to the lesser acuity. There is about 2 D of astigmatism at birth (initially against the rule and then with the rule) [38, 39]. The density of cones at the fovea of an infant is 1/4th of an adult and further the density of synapses in the neural portion of the retina as well as in the centres processing visual information in the brain, is low at birth [40, 41]. Also, there is poor myelination of nerves transmitting visual information leading to poor insulation of transmitted impulse.

1.5.2 Colour Vision and Contrast Sensitivity

Evaluating these visual functions in infants and early childhood remains a challenge. It is believed that at 3 months infants have dichromatic vision and have 1/50th of adult contrast sensitivity [42, 43]. By 4–6 months of age, they can distinguish between the primary colours [44].

1.5.3 Depth Perception

Stereopsis is absent at 3 months of age and believed to rapidly develop to normal levels by 6 months, exceeding the rate of development of visual acuity [45]. Hence the period between 3 and 6 months is critical. Accurate reaching behaviour develops in children between 5 and 13 months of age and it evolves to adult-like timing and accuracy by 8–9 years of age [46, 47]. By 2 years of age, children develop reasonable eye–hand coordination [48].

1.6 Emmetropization

It is the developmental process that balances the optical power of the eye and its axial length to focus the unaccommodated eye at distance [49]. Coordinated growth of the cornea, lens and the eyeball (axial length) with optical media clarity, genetic factors and the visual surroundings determine the refractive outcome in early years of development.

The overall refraction of the eye is mildly hyperopic at birth which initially increases and then undergoes a myopic shift towards emmetropia at around 7 years of age until the adult dimensions are reached at about 16 years of age [2]. In normal eyes growth of ocular structures is so coordinated that while the axial length increases significantly from birth to adulthood, the refraction changes minimally due to compensation by changes in the cornea and crystalline lens [27]. This compensation is lost in aphakic and pseudophakic eyes resulting in significant myopic shift. The changes in normal eyes have been listed below:

1. The refractive power of the cornea which is approximately 52 D (Dioptre) at birth which reduces to 44 D by 2 years of age, implying its flattening. The increase in corneal diameter from 8.5 mm at 34th week of gestation to 9.5 mm at birth and 11–12 mm in adults correlates with this physiological flattening [50].

2. The approximate power of the crystalline lens is 45 D which reduces by 20 D at 6 years [51, 52]. In preschool children, the range of accommodation is 20 D enabling them to focus despite the ongoing changes.
3. The axial length at birth is about 15.5–16.0 mm approximately, which increases to 20 mm at 1 year [53]. This increase occurs due to stretching and weakening of sclera governed by the intra-ocular pressure and action of metalloproteinase enzymes on scleral collagen [54]. By 6 years of age, the axial length increases by 5–6 mm to compensate for the loss of power of crystalline lens occurring during the same time frame. *In general, 1 mm change in axial length correlates with a 3-dioptre change in refractive power of eye* [55].

It is believed that the sharpness of image formed on the retina controls these changes. Understanding this phenomenon and being able to predict it is important for calculating the power of intra-ocular lens (IOL) at different ages.

1.7 Development of Binocular Single Vision

Frontal positioning of eyes during development leads to overlapping of visual fields. Consequently, an object is viewed simultaneously by both eyes. The goal of the entire process involving postnatal growth is to achieve binocular single vision, which is the hallmark of a fully developed visual system. In addition to anatomical alterations occurring in the eyes and the optical system to ensure a sharp image formation, motor and sensory alignment between eyes is equally important for maturation of cortical processes and development of binocularity.

With the consolidation of neural connections between visual cortex and eye, retinal locations in each eye share a common subjective visual direction in space. These retinal points in each eye are called ***Corresponding Retinal Points*** and any object's image falling upon them is perceived as a single object [56]. Typically, foveae of both eyes correspond with each other and are the carrier of the ***principal visual direction*** [57]. Not only is fovea the most differentiated retinal point with maximum cone density providing the best visual acuity, it is also considered as the seat for visual fixation [58]. Thus, in order for an object to be perceived as one, it is necessary that the visual axes (line joining fovea with the object of regard) of the eyes are aligned and image is formed over corresponding retinal points. This alignment is ensured by a fusional mechanism involving cortical unification of two visual images from each eye into a single image.

The development of 'vergence movement' by 3 months after birth allows for similar retinal images to be maintained on corresponding retinal points despite the tendency of natural (heterophorias) or artificial (prisms) causes to induce disparities. This phenomenon, termed as ***Motor Fusion***, refers to the ability to align the eyes in such a manner that sensory fusion can be maintained. ***Sensory Fusion*** is based upon the innate, orderly topographic relationship between the retina and the visual cortex, whereby images falling on corresponding retinal points in each eye are combined to form a single visual percept. At the same time, due to slight angle between the visual axes, there is always some horizontal disparity in images perceived by each eye. This disparity produces a subjective ordering of the visual object in depth or in three dimensions accounting for ***Stereopsis***. This is the ultimate level of visual development. Robust formation of cortical connections between eyes during the early phases of visual development in newborn is necessary to achieve binocular single vision and stereopsis. Congenital or developmental cataract can severely hamper this process of visual maturation and binocular interaction leading to suboptimal visual development in a child.

1.8 Amblyopia

vonNoorden defines amblyopia as '*decrease of visual acuity in one eye when caused by abnormal binocular interaction or occurring in one or both eyes as a result of pattern vision deprivation during visual immaturity, for which no cause can be detected during physical examination of the eye(s) and which in appropriate cases is reversible by therapeutic measures*' [59].

Pediatric cataract causes both vision deprivation and abnormal binocular interaction (in unilateral cataract) [60]. It is thus responsible for a profound amblyopia. Important discoveries in neurobiology have revealed the importance of visual stimulation in development of the visual pathways and concluded the following [61, 62]:

1. There is a critical period of visual development lasting a few weeks after birth which requires a normal postnatal visual stimulation. On basis of animal studies it is known, that the normally developed visual cortex has some cells driven by left and right eye individually but mostly the cells have binocular input. If one eye is deprived of visual stimulus, the cortex develops only cells connected to the non-deprived eye causing amblyopia of the deprived eye.
2. Changes in the visual cortex deprived of stimulation are partially or completely reversible by forced use of the deprived eye, if done correctly during the critical period of early childhood. It is believed that the critical period for visual rehabilitation extends well beyond the critical period for visual development forming the basis of occlusion therapy in amblyopia.
3. Cortical areas connected to the visually deprived eye shrink relative to the areas controlled by the normal fellow eye, suggesting some form of competition between the eyes for cortical space during the critical period.

Thus, it has been demonstrated that congenital cataract is not an irreversible cause of visual impairment provided timely surgery and rehabilitation are carried out during the critical period. The prevention and management of amblyopia have been covered in later chapters. It suffices here to say that media clarity should be restored within the critical period of development which is 6 weeks of birth for unilateral cataract and up to 14 weeks for bilateral cataracts [63, 64].

1.9 Congenital Abnormalities

The development and differentiation of the eye is a well-orchestrated and meticulous process. In spite of this, certain chromosomal abnormalities, environmental factors, and gene mutations play a causative role in developmental anomalies. Various congenital abnormalities of human eye can be grouped as under [65]:

(a) Agenesis—failure of development (e.g. anophthalmia).
(b) Hypoplasia—developmental arrest (e.g. optic nerve hypoplasia).
(c) Hyperplasia—excess development(e.g. distichiasis).
(d) Dysraphia—fusion failure (e.g. coloboma of choroid).
(e) Canalization failure—non-canalization (e.g. congenital nasolacrimal duct obstruction).
(f) Vestigial structure persistence—non-regression (e.g. persistent fetal vasculature).
(g) Maldevelopment—(e.g. Congenital cataract)

1. Anophthalmia is the absence of ocular tissue in one or both orbits. As a monogenic cause, the SOX2 gene has been implicated as a major causative gene. The environmental factors related to anophthalmia are viral infections (e.g. rubella), vitamin A deficiency, X-ray or thalidomide exposure during pregnancy [66].
2. Microphthalmia is presence of the axial length of an eye below 2 standard deviations of population adjusted mean, which in an adult eye is typically less than 21 mm. It is usually unilateral and associated with maternal age above 40 years, multiple childbirths, low birth weight or less gestational age [67].

   Nanophthalmos can be considered as a subtype, which is commonly bilateral and the eyes are evidently normal except for the small size. Microcornea, axial length below 18 mm and high hypermetropia ($\geq$8 D) are usual features [46]. The crystalline lens is normal in size making the anterior chamber very shallow. Any intra-ocular surgery is a challenge in these eyes and prone to complications.
3. Coloboma is caused by the failure of fusion of embryonic fissure during seventh week of embryonic life. The closure of the fissure first occurs at the centre and then progresses anteriorly and posteriorly in a 'zip' closure fashion. Most common structure affected is iris (Fig. 1.10). PAX2 and PAX6 are the commonly associated mutations. A typical coloboma is located inferonasally. The popular Ida Mann's classification of retino-choroidal colobomas is represented in the diagram (Fig. 1.17) [68, 69].
4. Optic nerve hypolplasia is the most frequent congenital anomaly of optic nerve head which may be unilateral or bilateral [70]. The typical tetrad associated with optic nerve hypoplasia is vascular tortuosity, thinning of retinal nerve fibre layer, peripapillary 'double ring sign' and small optic disc. Optic disc is abnormally small due to incomplete development of retinal ganglion cells resulting in decreased number of axons with the insult occurring in the first or early second trimester [71]. Common associations are endocrinopathies (hypopituitarism), developmental abnormalities and brain malformations.

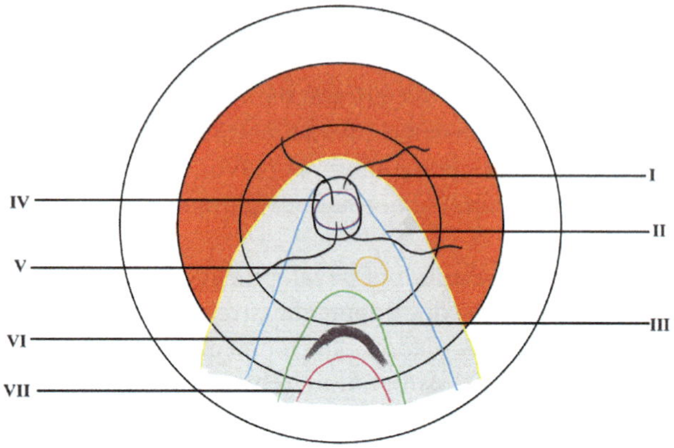

Fig. 1.17 Ida Mann's classification of retino-chorodial colobomas. The 7 types (I to VII) are based upon the location and extent of the defect

5. Persistent fetal vasculature (PFV) results due to anomalous or incomplete regression of the primary vascular vitreous together with abnormal increase in number (hyperplasia) of retinal astrocytes and optic nerve head glial cells. Earlier it was known as persistent hyperplastic primary vitreous (PHPV). It is usually unilateral, however, slight malformations may occur in the fellow eye [72]. It significantly impairs vision and may be classified as anterior, posterior or mixed depending on the region of vitreous involved [73].

   Anterior or mixed PFV may be associated with cataract and microphthalmia. It may present as leucocoria with retinoblastoma as an important differential diagnosis. The persistent hyaloid artery may cause troublesome bleeding during vitrectomy or posterior capsulotomy performed during pediatric cataract surgery.
6. Congenital cataract involving the embryonic nucleus occurs due to opacification of primary lens fibres. This is either due to failure of lengthening or aligning of these fibres in the earlier described organized manner [74]. Sutural cataract occurs following damage to secondary fibres. Congenital cataract may occur due to insult by viruses like rubella in the first trimester of pregnancy as primary lens fibres develop at this time. Etiology of congenital cataract is discussed in the next chapter.
7. Congenital opacity of cornea has diverse etiologies. Congenital corneal opacities are related to dystrophies of cornea, congenital glaucoma, dermoids, dysgenesis of anterior segment, birth trauma, microphthalmia, Axenfeld-Rieger syndrome etc. They are generally recognized by their morphology and location (central or peripheral, diffuse or localized and unilateral or bilateral). The most common treatment strategy for visually significant opacities is penetrating keratoplasty.
8. Congenital glaucoma commonly occurs due to dysgenesis of the trabecular meshwork. The eye may be enlarged due to scleral stretching by raised IOP resulting in Buphthalmos. Blepharospasm, photophobia and lacrimation are frequent symptoms. Haab striae form in the descemet membrane due to its stretching caused by oedema of corneal stroma. Goniotomy or trabeculectomy are common surgical procedures done for management.

1.10 Summary

- Embryogenesis, organogenesis and differentiation are the three cardinal steps in the development of embryo.
- Three primary germ layers called the ectoderm, mesoderm and endoderm are formed during the stage of gastrulation.
- The ocular tissues differentiate from ectoderm and mesoderm. Neuroectoderm, cranial neural crest cells and surface ectoderm form most of the structures.
- The crystalline lens develops from an indentation in the surface ectoderm called lens pit. The pit pinches off to form the lens vesicle, which after obliteration of central cavity develops into the crystalline lens.
- During growth of normal eyes from birth to adulthood the axial length increases significantly but the refraction changes minimally due to compensation by changes in the cornea and crystalline lens. This process is called emmetropization.
- Development and growth of the eye is a carefully balanced process. Any deviation from normal results in anomalies.

Acknowledgements The authors acknowledge the support of Mr. Ritwik Srivastava and Mr. Amit Mohan Yadav for designing the figures of this chapter.

Multiple Choice Questions

1. Which of the following structures is derived from cranial neural crest cells:
   (a) Retina
   (b) Conjunctival epithelium
   (c) Lens
   (d) Trabecular meshwork

   Answer: *d. Trabecular meshwork.* Retina is derived from neuroectoderm while lens and conjunctival epithelium are derived from surface ectoderm.

2. Which of the following is the correct sequence in the formation of crystalline lens:
   (a) Lens pit—lens vesicle—lens plate—lens
   (b) Lens plate—lens pit—lens vesicle—lens
   (c) Lens vesicle—lens pit—lens plate—lens
   (d) Lens plate—lens vesicle—lens pit—lens

   Answer: *b. Lens plate—lens pit—lens vesicle—lens.* Lens plate is the demarcation of region of presumptive lens on the surface ectoderm. Its indentation is called lens pit and when it pinches off it results in the formation of lens vesicle. Obliteration of its cavity results in the formation of the crystalline lens.

3. Which of the following is *incorrectly* matched:
   (a) Dysraphia—coloboma
   (b) Hyperplasia—distichiasis
   (c) Hypoplasia—persistent fetal vasculature
   (d) Agenesis—anophthalmia

   Answer: *c. Hypoplasia—persistent fetal vasculature.* Persistent fetal vasculature is an example of the failure of vestigial structures to regress.

4. Identify the most appropriate statement about emmetropization:
   (a) It is complete by 6 years of age.
   (b) Axial length increases, power of crystalline lens decreases and power of cornea increases.
   (c) Axial length increases, power of crystalline lens increases and power of cornea decreases.
   (d) Axial length increases, power of crystalline lens decreases and power of cornea decreases.

   Answer: *d. Axial length increases, power of crystalline lens decreases and power of cornea decreases.* Axial length increases from about 16 mm at birth to about 24 mm in adults. Power of cornea decreases from about 50 D at birth to about 44 D in adults and power of lens decreases from about 40 D at birth to about 20 D in adults. The process continues till about 16 years of age.

5. In regard to the development of crystalline lens, which of the following statement is *false*:
   (a) The oldest fibres represent the embryonic nucleus.
   (b) Mitotically active lens epithelial cells are at the equator and along the posterior capsule.
   (c) By identifying the zone of involvement in congenital cataract it is possible to have an idea of the time of insult.
   (d) It is derived from surface ectoderm.

   Answer: *b. Mitotically active lens epithelial cells are at the equator and along the posterior capsule.* The mitotically active cells are at the lens equator and anterior to it. There is no epithelium on the posterior capsule. By identifying the zone of involvement in zonular cataracts it is possible to identify the time of insult.

6. Which of the following statements is *incorrect* with regards to the differentiation of ocular structures:
   (a) Failure of lens vesicle separation from surface ectoderm causes keratolenticular adhesions.
   (b) Failure of fusion of embryonic fissure lips results in microphthalmia.

(c) Failure of regression of hyaloid system (primary vitreous) causes persistent fetal vasculature.
(d) Amblyopia causes cortical areas connected to the visually deprived eye to shrink relative to the areas controlled by the normal fellow eye.

Answer: *b. Failure of fusion of embryonic fissure lips results in microphthalmia.* Failure of fusion of embryonic fissure lips results in typical coloboma.

References

1. Ocular development. Fundamentals and principles of ophthalmology. American Academy of Ophthalmology. Vol. 2; 2015–2016. p. 111–27.
2. Growth and development of the eye. Paediatric ophthalmology and strabismus. American Academy of Ophthalmology. Vol. 6; 2015–2016. p. 181–7.
3. Ocular development. Fundamentals and principles of ophthalmology. American Academy of Ophthalmology. Vol. 2; 2009–2010. p. 113–43.
4. Cavodeassi F, Creuzet S, Etchevers HC. The hedgehog pathway and ocular developmental anomalies. Hum Genet. 2019;138(8–9):917–36.
5. Naderali E, Khaki AA, Rad JS, Ali-Hemmati A, Rahmati M, Charoudeh HN. Regulation and modulation of PTEN activity. Mol Biol Rep. 2018;45(6):2869–81.
6. Rose CF. Optic atrophy. Postgrad Med J. 1964;40:692.
7. Mann I. The early stages of the formation of the primary optic vesicle. The development of the human eye. 2nd ed; 1950. p. 1–15.
8. Mann I. A general outline of the development of optic vesicle and the associated mesoderm. The development of the human eye. 2nd ed; 1950. p. 16–45.
9. Barishak Y. Embryology of the eye and its adnexa. Switzerland: Karger; 2001.
10. Ozanics V, Rayborn M, Sagun D. Observation on the morphology of the developing primate cornea: epithelium, its innervations and anterior stroma. J Morphol. 1977;153:263–97.
11. Ozanics V, Rayborn M, Sagun D. Some aspects of corneal and sclera differentiation in the primate. Exp Eye Res. 1976;22:305–27.
12. Bron AJ, Tripathi R, Tripathi BJ. Development of the human eye. Wolff's anatomy of the eye and orbit. 8th ed; 1997. p. 621–64.
13. Cvekl A, Tamm ER. Anterior eye development and ocular mesenchyme: new insights from mouse models and human diseases. Bioessays. 2004;26:374–86.
14. Stiemke MM, Mccartney MD, Cantu-Croutch D, Edelhauser HF. Maturation of the corneal endothelial tight junction. Invest Ophthalmol Vis Sci. 1991;32:2757–65.
15. Steimke MM, Edelhauser HF, Geroski DH. The developing corneal endothelium: correlation of morphology, hydration and Na/k ATPase pump site density. Curr Eye Res. 1991;10:145–56.
16. Hogan M, Alvarado J, Wedell J. Histology of the human eye. Philadelphia: WB Saunders; 1971.
17. Dawson DG, Ubels JL, Edelhauser HF. Cornea and sclera. Adler's physiology of the eye. 11th ed; 2011. p. 71–125.
18. Tripathi BJ, Tripathi RC. Neural crest origin of the human trabecular meshwork and its implication for the pathogenesis of glaucoma. Am J Ophthalmol. 1989;230:583–90.
19. Foets B, van den Oord J, Engelmann K, et al. A comparative immunohistochemical study of human corneotrabecular tissue. Graefes Arch Clin Exp Ophthalmol. 1992;230:269–74.
20. Anderson DR. The development of the trabecular meshwork and its abnormality in primary infantile glaucoma. Trans Am Ophthalmol Soc. 1981;79:458–85.
21. Mann I. Vitreous and the sensory ligament of the lens. The development of the human eye. 2nd ed; 1950. p. 150–88.
22. The eye. Fundamentals and principles of ophthalmology. American Academy of Ophthalmology. Vol. 2; 2009–2010. p. 41–85.

23. Mann I. The neural ectoderm. The development of the human eye. 2nd ed; 1950. p. 68–149.
24. Tucker S, Jones B, Collin R. Systemic anomalies in 77 patients with congenital anophthalmos or microphthalmos. Eye. 1996;10:310–4.
25. Strouthidis NG, Papadopoulos M. Clinical evaluation of glaucoma in children. Curr Ophthalmol Rep. 2013;1:106–12.
26. Tucker SM, Sapp N, Collin R. Orbital expansion of the congenitally anophthalmic socket. Br J Ophthalmol. 1995;79:667–71.
27. Gordon RA, Donzis PB. Refractive development of human eye. Arch Ophthalmol. 1985;103(6):785–9.
28. Doughty MJ, Zaman ML. Human corneal thickness and its impact on intraocular pressure measures; a review and a metanalysis approach. Surv Ophthalmol. 2004;4:367–408.
29. Doughty MJ, Laiquzzaman M, Muller A, et al. Central corneal thickness in European(white) individuals, especially children and the elderly, and assessment of its possible importance in clinical measures of intraocular pressure. Ophthalmol Physiol Optics. 2002;22:491–504.
30. Avetisov S, Savitskaya N, Vinetskaya M, Imodina E. A study of biochemical and biomechanical qualities of normal and myopic eye sclera in human beings of different age groups. Metab Pediatr Syst Ophthalmol. 1983;7:183–8.
31. Grand IJ, Neely W, Sampson WG. The use of alpha chymotrypsin in infants and children. Am J Ophthalmol. 1962;54:95–101.
32. Raizman MB. Prolonged intraocular inflammation. Cataract surgery. 3rd ed; 2015. p. 687–91.
33. Childhood Glaucomas: Clinical presentation. Shields textbook of glaucoma. 6th ed; 2011. p. 218–43.
34. Zetterström C. Intraocular lens implantation in the pediatric eye. J Cataract Refract surg. 1997;23:559–600.
35. Hejtmancik JF, Piatigorsky J. Lens protein and their molecular biology. Albert and Jakobiec's principles and practice of ophthalmology, vol. 1. 3rd ed; 2008. p. 1341–64.
36. Brown AM. Development of visual sensitivity to light and color vision in human infants: a critical review. Vision Res. 1990;30(8):1159–88.
37. Almoqbel FM, Irving EL, Leat SJ. Visual acuity and contrast sensitivity development in children: sweep visually evoked potential and psychophysics. Optom Vis Sci. 2017;94:830–7.
38. Mohundra I, et al. Astigmatism in infants. Science. 1978:202–329.
39. Howland HC, et al. Astigmatism measured by photorefraction. Science. 1978:202–331.
40. Boothe RG, Dobson V, Teller DY. Postnatal development of vision in human and non human primates. Ann Rev Neurosci. 1985;8:495.
41. Reynolds CR, Fletcher F, Janzen E. Handbook of clinical child neurophysiology. New York: Plenum Press; 1989.
42. Werner JS, Wooten BR. Human infant colour vision and colour perception. Infant Behav Dev. 1979;2:241–73.
43. Brown A, Lindsey D. Contrast insensitivity: the critical immaturity in infant visual performance. Optometry Vision Sci. 2009;1986:572–6.
44. Polikanina RI. Development of color vision in newborn infants. Neurosci Behav Physiol. 1969;3:41–9.
45. Held R. What can rates of development tell us about underlying mechanisms? In: Granud C, editor. Visual perception and cognition in infancy. Erlbaum: Hillsdale, NJ; 1993. p. 75.
46. vonHofsten C. Action in development. Dev Sci. 2007;10(1):54–60.
47. vonHofsten C, Rönnqvist L. Preparation for grasping an object: a developmental study. J Exp Psychol Hum Percept Perform. 1988;14(4):610–21.
48. American Optometry Association; Infant vision: birth to 24 months of age @ 2020.
49. Troilo D, Smith EL, Nickla DL, Ashby R, Tkatchenko AV, Ostrin LA, et al. IMI – Report on experimental models of emmetropization and myopia. Invest Ophthalmol Vis Sci. 2019;60(3):M31–88.
50. Tucker SM, et al. Corneal diammeter axial length and intraocular pressure in premature infants. Ophthalmol. 1992;99:1296.
51. Murti DO, et al. Optical and structural development of crystalline lens in childhood. Invest Ophthalmol Vis Sci. 1997;39:120.

52. Wood ICL, Murti DO, Zadnik K. Crystalline lens parameters in infancy. Ophthalmol Physiol Opt. 1996;6:310.
53. Hussain RN, Shahid F, Woodruff G. Axial length in apparently normal pediatric eyes. Eur J Ophthalmol. 2014;24(1):120–3.
54. Larsen JS. The sagittal growth of eye. Ultrasonic measurement of axial length of the eye from birth to puberty. Actaophthalmology. 1971;49:872.
55. Schor P, Miller D. Optics. Adler's physiology of the eye. 11th ed; 2011. p. 1–26.
56. Sensory physiology and pathology. Paediatric ophthalmology and strabismus. American Academy of Ophthalmology. Vol. 6; 2015–2016. p. 53–64.
57. von Noorden GK. Binocular vision and space perception. Binocular vision and ocular motility. 6th ed; 2002. p. 7–35.
58. Zeffren BS, Applegate RA, Bradley A, van Heuven WA. Retinal fixation point location in the foveal avascular zone. Invest Ophthalmol Vis Sci. 1990;31:2099–105.
59. von Noorden GK. Mechanisms of amblyopia. Doc Ophthalmol. 1977;34:93.
60. Agrawal S, Singh N, Singh V. Non surgical management of strabismus. Strabismus for every ophthalmologist. 1st ed; 2019. p. 105–6.
61. Hubel DH. Exploration of the primary visual cortex, 1955–78. Nature. 1982;299:515–24.
62. Wiesel TN. Postnatal development of the visual cortex and the influence of environment. Nature. 1982;299:583–91.
63. Beller R, Hoyt CS, Marg E, et al. Good visual function after neonatal surgery for congenital monocular cataracts. Am J Ophthal. 1981;91:559–65.
64. Jacobson SG, Mohindra I, Held R. Development of visual acuity in infants with congenital cataracts. Br J Ophthal. 1981;65:727–35.
65. Jones KL, Jones MC, del Campo M. Smith's Recognizable patterns of human malformation. 7th ed. Philadelphia: Elsevier Saunders; 2013.
66. Verma AS, Fitzpatrick DR. Anophthalmia and microphthalmia. Orphanet J Rare Dis. 2007;2:47.
67. Bateman JB. Microphthalmos. Int Ophthalmol Clin. 1984;24(1):87–107.
68. Warburg M. Classsification of microphthalmos and coloboma. J Med Genet. 1993;30(8):664–9.
69. Mann IC. Developmental abnormalities of the eye. London: Cambridge University Press; 1937. p. 65–103.
70. Brodskey MC. Congenital disorders of the optic nerve: excavations and hypoplasia. Eye (Lond). 2004;18:1038–48.
71. Garcia-Fillon P, Borchert M. Prenatal determinants of optic nerve hypoplasia: review of suggested correlates and future focus. Surv Ophthalmol. 2013;58:610–9.
72. Reese AB. Persistent hyperplastic primary vitreous. Am J Ophthalmol. 1955;40(3):317–31.
73. Silbert M, Gunvood AS. Clinical review. Persistent hyperplastic primary vitreous. Clin Eye Vision Care. 2000;12(3–4):131–7.
74. Smelser GK. Embryology and morphology of the lens. Invest Ophthalmol. 1965;4:398.

Etiology of Pediatric Cataract

2

Rajat M. Srivastava, Ankita, and Siddharth Agrawal

2.1 Introduction

Pediatric cataracts have a diverse etiology. While most congenital cataracts are idiopathic, maternal infections, inherited disorders, and metabolic syndromes also account for a number of cases. In acquired cataracts, ocular trauma is the commonest cause. Understanding the etiology of pediatric cataract is important as cataract may be the presenting sign of many systemic and ocular diseases. Moreover, identifying the etiology helps in prognostication and optimum management of the cataract. Most of the congenital or developmental cataracts are bilateral but may be asymmetrical.

2.2 Epidemiology

In developing countries like India, pediatric cataract is among the commonest cause of childhood blindness accounting for up to 27% of all cases. Other common causes involve the cornea or the whole globe (microphthalmos, anophthalmos, trauma, etc.) [1]. It is the leading *treatable* cause of blindness in children with significant social impact in terms of disability-adjusted life years [2, 3]. The worldwide incidence ranges from 1.8 to 3.6/10,000 per year and the prevalence of pediatric cataract ranges from 0.42 to 2.05/10,000 in developed countries to 0.63–13.6/10,000 in developing ones [4, 5]. The wide range is not only because of difference in populations but also

R. M. Srivastava · S. Agrawal (✉)
Department of Ophthalmology, King George's Medical University, Lucknow, India

Ankita
Department of Ophthalmology, Ganesh Shankar Vidyarthi Memorial Medical College, Kanpur, India

S. Agrawal (ed.), *Pediatric Cataract*,
https://doi.org/10.1007/978-981-16-1736-2_2

due to variety of methods, definitions used and the age groups studied. Congenital cataracts are associated with ocular and systemic abnormalities in about 27% and 22% of cases, respectively [5]. Differences on basis of gender and laterality have not been reported [6]. The commonest presentation is with leukocoria or strabismus. Incidental diagnosis during screening is common in developed countries [7].

2.3 Pathophysiology

Congenital cataract is believed to be majorly caused due to anomalies in genetic processes involved in lens development. This may result in isolated lenticular opacities if the anomaly is limited to lens-specific proteins (crystallins) or a systemic syndromic association in presence of anomalies affecting the chromosomes (Down syndrome) [8, 9]. Abnormal lens proteins undergo aggregation and compromise lens transparency. In addition, mutations in master genes involved in eye development can cause cataract in association with other gross developmental defects of the eye. Besides genetic insult, nutritional deficiencies and oxidative damage to the growing lens fibers due to infections and inflammation can also affect normal lens development. Furthermore, enzymatic defects as seen in metabolic disorders can lead to the accumulation of metabolic byproducts in lens. This leads to osmotic failure and cataract formation [10].

Among acquired causes, damage to lens capsule following trauma can cause hydration of lens fibers or affect its metabolism leading to cataract development. Chronic inflammatory pathologies pose a prolonged demand on the anti-oxidative mechanisms and continued oxidative damage along with depletion of antioxidants lead to cataract. Long-term steroid use has been known to cause metabolic alterations and osmotic failure in lens. Formation of nonenzymatic steroid–lens protein complexes alter the solubility of lens proteins and result in lens opacification [11]. Thus, cataractogenesis is multifactorial and oxidative damage in addition to genetic and metabolic alterations have been implicated in cataract formation.

2.4 Genetics

As discussed in the previous chapter formation of lens placodes occurs at 28 days of gestation. Fibroblast growth factor (FGF) and bone morphogenetic protein are responsible for induction and formation of the lens. Mutations involving 40 genes encoding crystallins (e.g., CRYAA, CRYAB), cytoskeletal proteins (e.g., BFSP1), membrane proteins (connexin genes, e.g., GJA3), and transcription factors (e.g., PITX3) have been identified [5, 12]. These mutations are usually autosomal dominant (AD) and the timing of insult determines the lenticular part involved [13].

Congenital cataracts are hereditary, implying that the mutations are passed onto the next generation in 8–25% of cases, with 75% of these having AD inheritance [14]. However, a similar phenotype of cataract is observed in mutations of different genes while similar mutations of the same gene can result in different cataract phenotypes [15]. Thus, penetrance is variable. Examples of AD inheritance are cataracts associated with hyperferritinemia and myotonic dystrophy 1. Those of autosomal recessive inheritance are Warburg micro syndrome and Wilson disease and that of X-linked inheritance is Norrie disease [16, 17].

The deleterious manifestation of the mutations may be limited to a specific type of cataract (e.g., anterior polar cataract in PAX6 and posterior polar in PITX3 mutations) or may cause major syndromes associated with cataracts (e.g., Galactosemia in GALK117q and Lowe syndrome in OCRL) [18–20].

2.5 Etiology

Congenital cataract refers to any lenticular opacity present at birth, although it may also present in infancy. The laterality, location, and morphology of cataract may provide clues about the etiology of cataract and time of insult (Fig. 2.1, Tables 2.1 and 2.2).

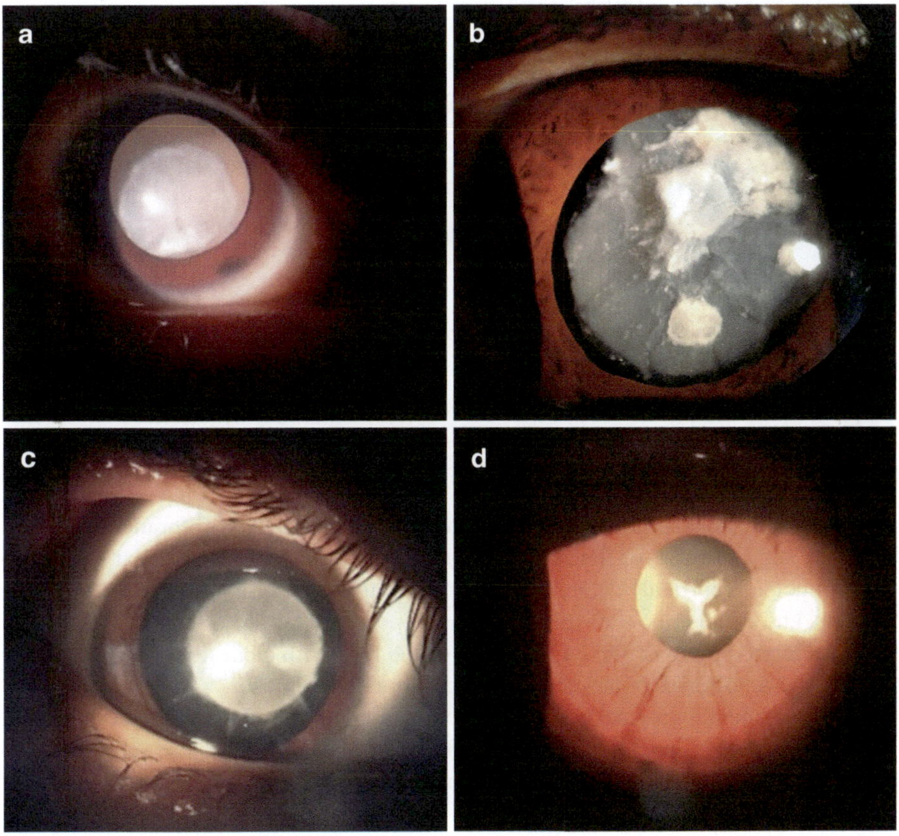

Fig. 2.1 Different morphological types of cataract in children. (**a**) Total cataract, (**b**) Dense nuclear (rubella) cataract, (**c**) Zonular or lamellar cataract with radial "rider" opacities, (**d**) Sutural cataract, (**e**) Posterior polar cataract, (**f**) Posterior subcapsular cataract, and (**g**) Cataract associated with aniridia. Vascularization is seen on the surface of the cataractous lens

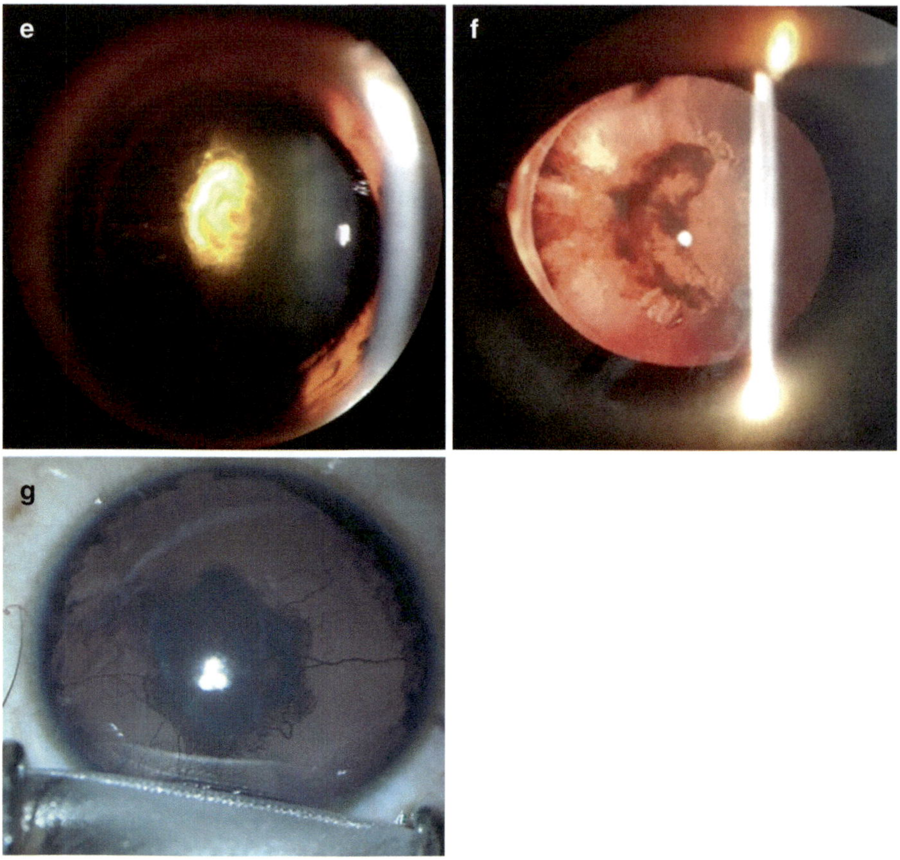

Fig. 2.1 (continued)

Embryonal nuclear (small central) cataract suggests insult during first 2 months of gestation, fetal nuclear (between level of anterior and posterior Y sutures) cataract is due to insult at about 3 months and sutural opacities with branching (arborization) suggest an even later insult during gestation [6, 8]. Lamellar (Zonular) or perinuclear (cortical) cataract is concentric to the lens capsule, surrounds the nucleus, and occurs due to insult occurring in perinatal period or early childhood. It is characterized by opacities in one layer of the lens with clear fibers on both sides. Anterior and posterior polar cataract suggest congenital onset.

"Developmental cataract" is used for congenital and infantile cataracts together. Acquired cataracts in children develop following any insult to lens, either due to trauma (traumatic), surgery (iatrogenic) or intraocular pathology (secondary) [6].

Table 2.1 Etiological classification of pediatric cataracts [21]

Bilateral cataracts	**Unilateral cataracts**
Idiopathic	Idiopathic
Maternal infections • Rubella, toxoplasma, cytomegalovirus, varicella, syphilis, herpes	Trauma
Metabolic and systemic disorders • Galactosemia, Wilson disease, Diabetes mellitus, Lowe Syndrome, Alport syndrome, Myotonic dystrophy	Secondary • Retinal detachment, uveitis
Ocular malformations/ocular syndromes • Anterior segment dysgenesis, aniridia	Ocular malformations/ocular syndromes • Persistent fetal vasculature (PFV), anterior segment dysgenesis
Chromosomal abnormality • Trisomy 21 (Down), Trisomy 13 (Patau), Trisomy 18 (Edward), Monosomy X (Turner)	Treatment induced (Iatrogenic) • Corticosteroid, radiation, post vitrectomy
Isolated hereditary (usually autosomal dominant)	
Treatment induced (Iatrogenic) • Corticosteroid, radiation, post vitrectomy	

Table 2.2 Characteristic morphological types of pediatric cataracts

Location of opacity	**Morphology**	**Possible etiology**	**Associated findings/ remarks**
Anterior			
Anterior polar	Small opacities on anterior surface of lens/pyramidal	Peters anomaly	Anterior segment dysgenesis, aniridia
Anterior subcapsular	Rosette	Blunt trauma	Vossius ring
	Sunflower (green)	Wilson disease	Kayser Fleischer (KF) ring
	Anterior lenticonus	Alport syndrome	Nephritis
Central (Cortical, Nuclear)			
Central	Oil droplet	Galactosemia	Mental retardation, jaundice
	Lamellar (Zonular)	Hereditary (AD)	Similar morphology of cataract also seen in children with rickets
	Thin disciform	Lowe syndrome	Hypotonia, glaucoma
Cortical	Blue dot opacities, pulverulent/cerulean, and coronary	Hereditary/ metabolic	Blue dot opacities are usually insignificant visually
	Christmas tree (multicolored flecks)	Myotonic dystrophy	Ophthalmoplegia, retinopathy, cataract may even be subcapsular
Sutural	Along Y suture	Nance Horan carriers [22]	Retinitis Pigmentosa, microcephaly, developmental delay [23]

(continued)

Table 2.2 (continued)

Location of opacity	Morphology	Possible etiology	Associated findings/ remarks
Peripheral			
	Vacuolar	Prematurity	Visually insignificant, resolve with time
Posterior			
Posterior polar	Posterior capsule plaque	Persistent fetal vasculature syndrome	Mittendorf dot, high myopia
Posterior subcapsular	Vacuolar	Diabetes mellitus	Diabetic retinopathy
	Spoke like	Fabry syndrome	Cornea verticillata (whorls)
	Posterior lenticonus (congenital thinning and bowing of posterior capsule, later opacification)	Autosomal recessive inheritance	Oil droplet reflex on retinoscopy, may also be associated with Lowe syndrome
Total/diffuse			
Central total	Dense complete opacification	Rubella	Microphthalmia, coloboma. May also be due to metabolic disorders or trauma
Partially Absorbed	Membranous	Hallerman-Francois syndrome	Microphthalmos, brachycephaly, beak-like nose, micrognathia. May also occur in trauma

2.5.1 Idiopathic

More than 50% of congenital cataracts are idiopathic [24]. Low birth weight, multiple pregnancies, placental insufficiency, respiratory distress, maternal preeclampsia, use of certain drugs during pregnancy have been associated with congenital cataract. Exhaustion of glutathione due to prenatal oxidative stress may explain a possible association between maternal malnutrition, low birth weight, and idiopathic cataract [25]. Environmental stress can also act as a trigger in genetically predisposed cases. Although several mechanisms have been proposed, cataractogenesis in several cases still remains poorly understood; indicating a possible multifactorial origin [26, 27].

2.5.2 Maternal Infections

Maternal infection during the first trimester affects fetuses more severely, however, fetal transmission is more frequent in last trimester [28].

Cataract occurs secondary to maternal transmission of toxoplasma, rubella, cytomegalovirus, herpes simplex, varicella zoster and syphilis (TORCH). Rubella is the commonest in developing countries. Infections acquired during first trimester, result in influx of the virus into the developing primary lens fibers through hyaloid vessels. This interferes with the lenticular protein synthesis causing in utero lens opacification. The persistence of virus in lens also causes subsequent metabolic disturbances explaining development of cataract later during infancy. Last trimester infections rarely reach the lens, but can still result in cataract because of metabolic disturbances induced by vasculitis [29]. Secondary cataract is associated with infections causing anterior segment inflammation of the eye [25, 30, 31]. Characteristic features of congenital cataract and associated systemic abnormalities in children related to intrauterine transmission of various maternal infections resulting in cataract are elucidated in Table 2.3. They are usually bilateral and present at birth, however, onset may be delayed till 1 year of age.

Table 2.3 Cataracts associated with Maternal Infections

Maternal infection	Type of cataract	Ocular features	Systemic features
Rubella (commonest in developing countries)	Nuclear, total (density is variable and depends on viral load in fibers) [5]	Microphthalmos, salt, and pepper retinopathy	Cardiac disorders (commonly patent ductus arteriosus), sensorineural hearing loss, hepatosplenomegaly, mental retardation
Varicella	Nuclear [32]	Microphthalmos, chorioretinitis, and optic atrophy [33]	Cicatricial skin scarring, microcephaly, seizure, mental retardation, renal abnormalities
Herpes simplex (HSV-2 infection is commoner than HSV-1)	Nuclear/lamellar (maybe secondary following neonatal infection)	Chorioretinitis (conjunctivitis and keratitis may occur in neonatal infection) [34]	Mucocutaneous lesions, seizures, focal neurological signs, respiratory distress, acute liver failure
Cytomegalovirus (commonest in developed countries)	Nuclear/lamellar	Retinitis, optic disc and anterior chamber malformations, microphthalmos, strabismus [26]	Mental retardation, microcephaly, sensorineural hearing loss
Toxoplasmosis	Nuclear/lamellar (usually secondary to inflammation) [35]	Chorioretinitis, iridocyclitis, retinal detachment, nystagmus, strabismus	Seizures, microcephaly, hydrocephalus, cerebral calcification, psychomotor retardation, jaundice
Syphilis	Nuclear/lamellar (may be secondary to inflammation)	Salt and pepper retinopathy, uveitis, interstitial keratitis, optic atrophy, and rarely eyelid chancres	Deafness (Cranial Nerve VIII), Hutchinson teeth (notched incisors), Clutton joints (painless swelling of joints), saddle nose, frontal bossing vesico bullous skin eruptions, seizures, mental retardation

2.5.3 Metabolic and Systemic Disorders

Metabolic and systemic disorders associated with cataracts have varied inheritance. The cataract is usually bilateral and often has a characteristic appearance. The children have multiple system involvement and cataract is usually not the presenting symptom. Frequently seen metabolic disorders associated with cataract are listed in Table 2.4.

Table 2.4 Metabolic and systemic disorders associated with cataracts in children

Metabolic disorder	Inheritance	Age of onset	Type of cataract	Systemic features
Galactosemia	Autosomal recessive	Newborn (may manifest up to adulthood)	Oil droplet, nuclear, subcapsular, lamellar (Cataract is initially reversible) [36]. Milder cataract occurs in galactokinase deficiency	Mental retardation, failure to thrive hepatomegaly, splenomegaly, and jaundice [37]
Diabetes mellitus	Sporadic	Childhood-adolescence	Anterior or posterior subcapsular, snowflake	Cardiovascular renal, neurological abnormalities
Hypoparathyroidism	X-linked recessive	Childhood-adolescence	Lamellar with discrete opacities (may be transient, usually visually insignificant) [31]	Hypocalcemia, seizures, muscle pain and craps, soft teeth, dry skin, patchy alopecia, and mental retardation
Glucose-6-phosphate dehydrogenase deficiency	X-linked recessive	Childhood-adolscence	Total	Mental and psychomotor disorders, seizures, and anemia
Alport syndrome	Autosomal dominant	Late childhood	Anterior lenticonus, lamellar	Familial hemorrhagic nephritis, nerve deafness
Wilson disease	Autosomal recessive	Adolescence	Anterior/ posterior capsular, anterior polar, ray-like lenticular opacities (sunflower)	Hepatic, neuropsychiatric, Osseo muscular, hematological renal

Table 2.4 (continued)

Metabolic disorder	Inheritance	Age of onset	Type of cataract	Systemic features
Lowe syndrome (oculo-cerebral-renal syndrome)	X-linked recessive	Birth/infancy	Nuclear (disciform), total, posterior polar	Mental and psychomotor retardation, short stature, frontal bossing, aminoaciduria, vitamin D-resistant rickets
Norrie disease	X-linked recessive	Neonate to infancy	Dense total cataract	Early childhood blindness (retinal detachment, vitreous hemorrhage), sensorineural deafness, developmental delay

2.5.4 Ocular Malformations

Cataract may be associated with anterior segment dysgenesis like Peters anomaly, posterior embryotoxon, and microcornea and is mostly sporadic. Cataract is mostly nuclear or sometimes anterior polar. A pre-existing posterior capsular defect may be seen in association with a posterior polar cataract, persistent fetal vasculature (PFV), lenticonus, or lentiglobus. This may cause hydration of lens manifesting as a total cataract or merely a white spot on posterior lens capsule and is confirmed by ultrasound biomicroscopy (UBM) [5, 38].

PFV earlier known as persistent hyperplastic primary vitreous (PHPV) occurs due to anomalous or incomplete regression of the primary vascular vitreous and is one of the commonest causes of unilateral cataract in infants [39]. The pathogenesis of PFV has been discussed in the previous chapter. It is an isolated, sporadic, unilateral malformation causing the affected eye to be smaller than normal in size. It may rarely be bilateral when it is associated with systemic abnormalities.

PFV has a wide spectrum of severity. Mild PFV may be visually insignificant with the presence of prominence of hyaloid vessel remnants, Mittendorf dot (dense, circular opacity on posterior lens capsule), and Bergmeister papilla (fibrous tissue attached to the optic disc) [40]. Microphthalmos, thick fibrous persistent hyaloid artery with traction on optic disc, distortion of posterior retina, elongated ciliary processes, and dense retrolenticular plaque are features of severe PFV. Varying degrees of progressive cataract may occur, associated with anterior chamber shallowing and secondary glaucoma. Extreme cases may have ciliary body detachment, vitreous hemorrhage, congenital retinal nonattachment, and optic nerve dysmorphism [21].

It may be useful to recall here that severe PFV may present as leukocoria with secondary glaucoma and may need to be differentiated from retinoblastoma. In this scenario, a small eye with presence of cataract is suggestive of PFV whereas an enlarged or normal-sized eyeball is usual in retinoblastoma.

2.5.5 Chromosomal Abnormalities

In a number of these syndromes, cataract develops within a few weeks or months of life, commonest being Down syndrome. Table 2.5 elucidates cataract associated with various chromosomal abnormalities.

2.5.6 Isolated Hereditary (Familial) Cataract

As has been discussed earlier, genetic abnormalities can be identified in almost half of congenital cataracts. These affect lens protein folding, solubility, packing, and organization. Cataract may be isolated or maybe a part of an ocular or systemic

Table 2.5 Cataracts associated with chromosomal abnormalities

Genetic disorder	Age of onset	Type of cataract	Systemic features
Down syndrome (Trisomy 21)	Birth to adulthood [41]	Arcuate, polar, lamellar	Growth retardation, mental retardation, umbilical hernia, congenital cardiac disorder (ASD/VSD/PDA/TOF), epilepsy, leukemia, typical Mongoloid facial features (flat head, flattened nose, upward slanting of eyes), single palmar crease, separation of first and second toes
Patau syndrome (Trisomy 13)	Birth [42, 43]	Variable	Heart defects (ASD/VSD), spinal cord abnormalities, mental retardation, growth failure, renal deformities, cleft lip, cleft palate, umbilical hernia, cryptorchidism, dysplastic/malformed ears, hypotonia, polydactyly
Edward syndrome (Trisomy 18)	Birth [44, 45]	Variable	Prominent occiput, cleft lip/palate, low set malformed ears, short sternum, overlapping fingers, rocker bottom feet, cardiac and renal malformation, developmental delays
Turner syndrome (Monosomy of second sex chromosome in females XO)	Variable(Birth/ puberty/ presenile) [46, 47]	Total	Short stature, gondal dysgenesis (streak ovaries), webbed neck, low hairline at back of neck, shield-shaped thorax, widely spaced nipples, cardiac abnormalities (coarctation of aorta/aortic valve abnormalities), developmental delays

syndrome. Those associated with syndromes have been discussed earlier. Non-syndromic (isolated) congenital cataract is described here.

Crystallin and connexin gene mutations are most frequent [48]. Autosomal dominant inheritance is the most common, followed by X-linked and autosomal recessive. Genes involved in cataractogenesis are expressed in a sequential manner during development.

Cataract morphology provides a clue about the underlying genotype and the time of insult. For example, EPHA2, PITX3, CRYAB genes on 1p, 10q, and 11q chromosomes have been identified for posterior polar cataract. Blue-dot (Cerulean) cataract is attributed to CRYBB2 gene on 22q and CRYGD gene on 2q chromosomes. It develops during childhood, progresses throughout life, and is visually insignificant [49, 50]. Similarly, genes have also been identified for Coppock (central pulverulent) cataract (CRYGC on 2q and CRYBB2 on 22q chromosome), hyperferritinemia cataract (FTL on 19q chromosome), and many others.

2.5.7 Traumatic Cataract

Trauma is a major cause of acquired cataracts in children. It is also the commonest cause of unilateral cataracts. The incidence is more common in males, rural areas, and penetrating trauma [22, 28, 51].

In penetrating injury, laceration of the lens capsule may initially cause a localized opacity which may remain stable but usually progresses to cataract formation in the entire lens. A focal rusty opacity called siderosis lentis may result from a retained intralenticular metallic foreign body [52].

Blunt trauma causes dysfunction of lens epithelium leading to edema of the superficial cortical fibers that may subsequently undergo degeneration and localized opacification. It may cause a typical rosette cataract [53]. Deposition of iris pigment over anterior lens capsule (Vossius ring) and disruption of lens zonular fibers causing dislocation or subluxation (partial disruption of fibers) are other lenticular characteristics of blunt trauma (Fig. 2.2).

Traumatic cataract and its management has been discussed in a later chapter.

2.5.8 Secondary and Iatrogenic Cataracts

This group includes cataract formed secondary to systemic causes like Juvenile idiopathic arthritis (JIA) and diabetes mellitus. Cataracts formed due to other pathologies in the eye like uveitis are classically called complicated cataracts [54]. Steroid use, radiation, or intraocular surgery can also result in cataract formation. Intraocular tumors and chronic retinal detachment also predispose to cataract formation [26].

Prevalence of cataract due to intraocular inflammation is 25–40% in children of uveitis [55, 56]. JIA is the commonest cause of uveitis and secondary cataract in children [5, 26]. Usual presentation is with posterior subcapsular opacity associated with posterior synechiae, iris bombe, and peripheral anterior synechiae. Band-shaped keratopathy and hypotony may occur in long-standing cases of JIA [52]. Cataract may also occur as a complication of chronic corticosteroid therapy used for its treatment. Both systemic and local steroids are used in management. Initially, dosage up to 10 mg/day of prednisone for 1 year was considered safe, however, cataract has been reported at lower doses (a cumulative dose of 1000 mg of prednisone or equivalent) in children leading to the concept that there is no really "safe" dose [11, 57]. Systemic immunosuppressive treatment is often recommended to eliminate the use of steroids and their adverse effects. However, it should be remembered that as immunosuppressive therapy may have serious and potentially life-threatening side effects, it should be initiated only in consultation with an immunologist and a pediatrician. Even after cataract surgery, JIA associated uveitis has poorer prognosis as compared to non-JIA uveitis (Fig. 2.3).

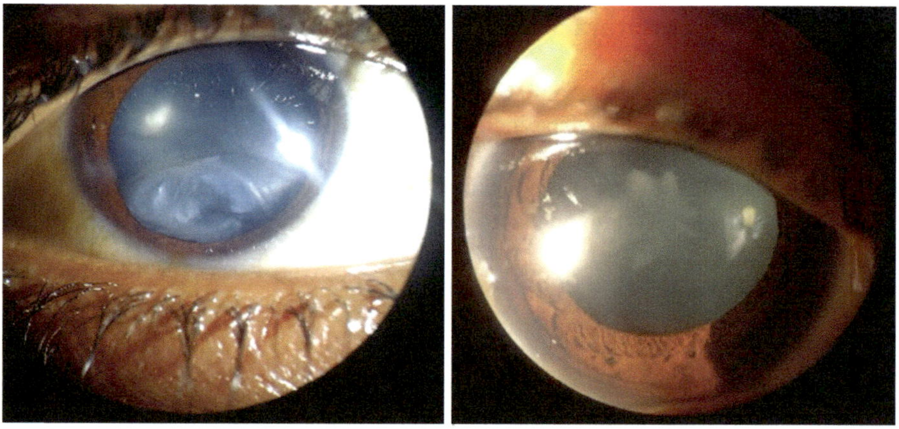

Fig. 2.2 Traumatic cataracts: Following penetrating injury (left) and rosette shaped after blunt injury (right) (Photograph courtesy: Dr. Ankur Yadav, Lucknow, India & Dr Rajat Kapoor, Hyderabad, India)

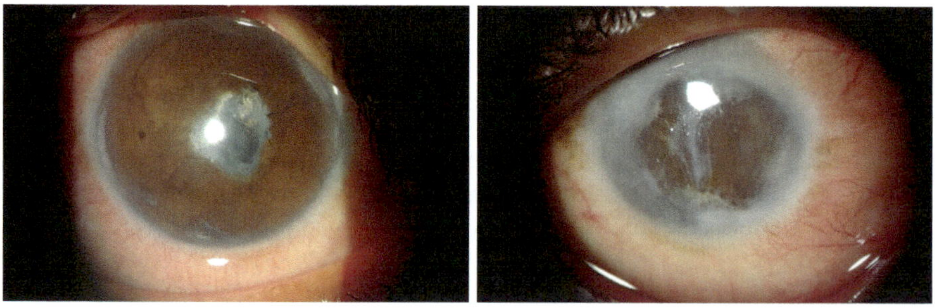

Fig. 2.3 Persistent inflammation with formation of pupillary membrane in a patient with Juvenile Idiopathic Arthritis (left) and phthisical other eye of the same patient (right)

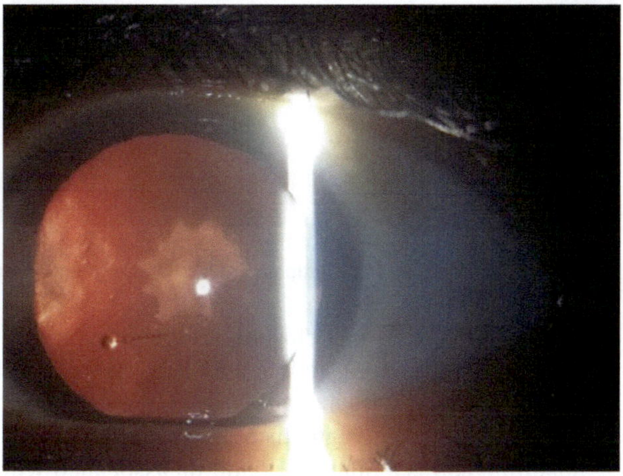

Fig. 2.4 Steroid-induced posterior subcapsular cataract

A cumulative radiation dose of 15 Gray is associated with 50% risk of cataract formation [22, 58]. The cataract formation may occur several years after the initial exposure or may occur suddenly after a large dose.

Secondary cataracts are commonly posterior subcapsular (Fig. 2.4). They are unilateral if the cause is local (e.g., localized radiation) and bilateral if the disease is generalized (e.g., diabetes mellitus, JIA). Iatrogenic cataracts are formed following vitrectomy or lasers for retinal diseases [26].

2.5.9 Cataract in Prematurity

Premature birth predisposes to cataract in neonates, though the exact cause of this is still poorly understood. They differ from other congenital cataracts as they arise peripherally, anterior to the posterior lens suture as clear vacuoles and are generally reversible; resolving within few weeks to months [22, 25].

2.6 Abnormalities in Structure and Position of the Crystalline Lens

In children, the crystalline lens may be occasionally structurally abnormal, subluxated, or dislocated without cataractous changes. These conditions need to be identified and managed timely to prevent complications.

2.6.1 Structural Abnormalities

Congenital aphakia is rare and is associated with a grossly abnormal eye.

Lens coloboma is actually a misnomer, as the lens appears colobomatous due to the absence or weakness of zonules. Typical colobomas are present inferonasally,

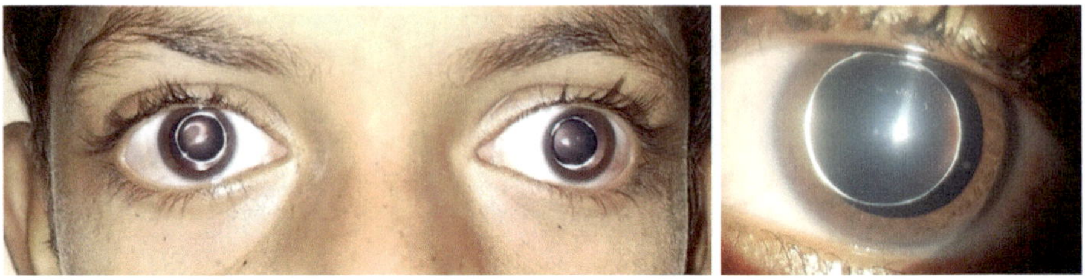

Fig. 2.5 Spherophakia (Photograph courtesy: Dr. Deepika Verma, Lucknow, India)

representing the abnormal closure of the embryonic fissure and may be associated with colobomas of uvea, retina, and optic nerve. As the defect is congenital and usually nonprogressive, management of a pure lens coloboma consists of optical correction of myopic astigmatism.

Spherophakia is a bilateral condition associated with lenses that are smaller and more spherical than normal. The primary abnormality is defective development of lens zonules and these abnormal lenses are prone to dislocation (Fig. 2.5).

Duplication of lens is a rare condition caused due to metaplastic change in surface ectoderm preventing the normal invagination of the lens placode and thereby resulting in formation of two lens vesicles. The condition is associated with uveal tissue coloboma and corneal metaplasia.

Lenticonus and lentiglobus are caused due to thinning of the lens capsule with deficiency of the epithelial cells resulting in abnormality of the lens curvature. In lenticonus the resultant protrusion of the lens surface is conical and localized whereas in lentiglobus it is spherical and usually involves the entire surface. Posterior lenticonus is commoner, inherited as autosomal recessive trait or may be associated with systemic abnormalities like oculo-cerebral syndrome of Lowe. Anterior lenticonus is associated with Alport syndrome. Both lenticonus and lentiglobus cause lenticular myopia with irregular astigmatism. An oil droplet reflex may be seen on retinoscopy. They are associated with opacification of posterior polar fibers causing polar cataract. Spontaneous or intraoperative rupture of the weak capsule may occur.

2.6.2 Positional Anomalies

Disruption of the zonules results in the lens moving away from its normal anatomical place known as *ectopia lentis*. Although the pathophysiology is same, yet based on severity, the lens is considered subluxated (if some zonules are intact and a part of the lens is in pupillary axis) or luxated/dislocated (if it is completely detached from the ciliary body). It is important to identify the cause of zonular disruption as some are progressive (e.g., Marfan syndrome, homocystinuria) while others are stationary (e.g., trauma). It would be safe to advise a systemic evaluation when zonular disruption is noticed in the absence of history of trauma (Fig. 2.6). However, a history of ocular trauma does not preclude other causes of ectopia lentis.

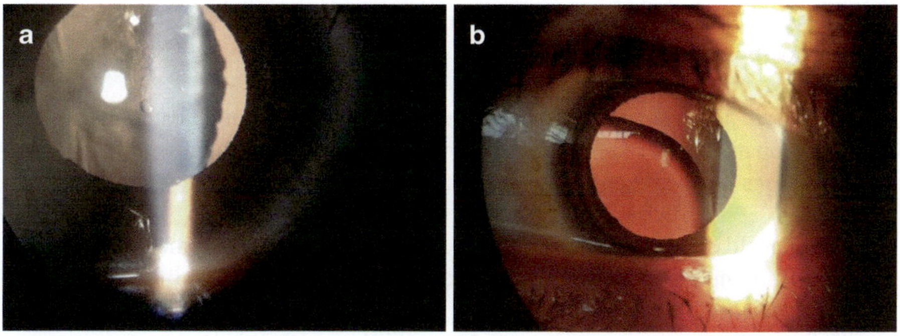

Fig. 2.6 (**a**) and (**b**) Increasing grades of non-traumatic subluxation of the crystalline lens. It is important to perform a systemic evaluation to determine the cause

Optical correction, though difficult, should be tried. When the subluxation is mild, correction of myopia or myopic astigmatism is done but when it is severe, aphakic correction often provides better visual quality. If optical correction does not provide satisfactory visual functions or the condition is progressive, lensectomy is indicated [21]. Examination of retinal periphery and laser barrage of suspicious lesions should be done preoperatively.

2.7 Summary

- Etiology of pediatric cataracts is diverse. Most cases are idiopathic.
- Congenital and developmental cataracts are usually bilateral but may be asymmetrical.
- Maternal TORCH infections are the commonest identifiable cause in developing nations. Rubella is the commonest infection among them.
- Type I diabetes is a common cause of metabolic (secondary) cataract in children.
- Family history may suggest an inherited cause of cataract. Pattern of inheritance in hereditary cataract is autosomal dominant.
- Certain morphological types may be suggestive of a particular etiology and certain etiologies may have specific morphological types of cataract, however, neither are exclusive.
- Down Syndrome (Trisomy 21) is commonly associated with early onset of cataract.
- Trauma is frequent and preventable cause of cataract in children.

Multiple Choice Questions

1. A 3-month-old child is diagnosed with congenital cataract. Which of the following statements is true about such cataracts:
   (a) More than 50% of cases are idiopathic
   (b) They are reversible

(c) Typically associated with ocular malformations
(d) Mostly Autosomal recessive

Answer: *a. More than 50% of cases are idiopathic.* Congenital cataracts are usually idiopathic. They are irreversible, only a few are associated with ocular malformations and are usually autosomal dominant.

2. A 1-year-old child presents with failure to thrive, hepatosplenomegaly, and jaundice. Slit lamp examination is most likely to reveal which type of cataract:
   (a) Posterior polar cataract
   (b) Sutural cataract
   (c) Rosette cataract
   (d) Oil droplet cataract

   Answer: *d. Oil droplet cataract.* The child is suffering from Galactosemia. Galactitol, the metabolic end product, is relatively less permeable across lens fiber membranes. Subsequent hydration of lens fibers results in classical oil-droplet cataract. Such cataracts, develop within few weeks after birth, are bilateral and usually reversible after withdrawal of galactose from diet.

3. Which of the following statements is true regarding cataract associated with growth retardation, mental retardation, and mongoloid features:
   (a) It is reversible
   (b) Associated with maternal rubella infection
   (c) Mostly sutural cataracts
   (d) May manifest from birth till infancy

   Answer: *d. May manifest from birth till infancy.* Down syndrome is associated with growth retardation, mental retardation, umbilical hernia, congenital cardiac disorder (ASD/VSD/PDA/TOF), and typical Mongoloid facial features (flat head, flattened nose, upward slanting of eyes). The cataract may manifest from birth to adulthood, and is usually arcuate, polar, or lamellar in morphology.

4. Which of the following is the commonest cause of pediatric cataract in developed countries:
   (a) Maternal rubella infection
   (b) Maternal HSV-1 infection
   (c) Intrauterine CMV infection
   (d) Congenital syphilis

   Answer: *c. Intrauterine CMV infection.* Maternal CMV infection is the commonest cause in developed countries, Rubella infection still remains the commonest in developing countries. Cataract in CMV infection is nuclear or lamellar, associated with mental retardation, microcephaly, and sensorineural hearing loss.

5. Which of the following is the most common cause of acquired cataract in the pediatric population:
   (a) Uveitis
   (b) Steroid induced
   (c) Traumatic
   (d) Intraocular surgery

   Answer: c. *Traumatic.* Trauma is the commonest cause of acquired cataracts in children. Traumatic cataract is commonly unilateral, occurs in rural areas and has male preponderance. Penetrating trauma is associated with cataract more frequently than blunt trauma.

6. Which of the following is true about congenital cataracts:
   (a) It is commoner in boys.
   (b) It is the leading treatable cause of blindness in children.
   (c) Left eye is commonly involved.
   (d) Commonest presenting symptom is decrease in vision.

   Answer: b. *It is the leading treatable cause of blindness in children.* Differences in gender and laterality have not been reported in congenital cataracts. The commonest presenting symptoms are leukocoria (white pupillary reflex) and strabismus.

References

1. Wadhwani M, Vashist P, Singh SS, Gupta V, Gupta N, Saxena R. Prevalence and causes of childhood blindness in India: a systematic review. Indian J Ophthalmol. 2020;68:311–5.
2. Gilbert C, Foster A. Childhood blindness in the context of VISION 2020–the right to sight. Bull World Health Organ. 2001;79(3):227–32.
3. Rahi JS, Sripathi S, Gilbert CE, Foster A. Childhood blindness in India: causes in 1318 blind school students in nine states. Eye (Lond). 1995;9(Pt 5):545–50.
4. Wu X, Long E, Lin H, Liu Y. Prevalence and epidemiological characteristics of congenital cataract: a systematic review and meta-analysis. Sci Rep. 2016;6:28564.
5. Khokhar SK, Pillay G, Dhull C, Agarwal E, Mahabir M, Aggarwal P. Pediatric cataract. Indian J Ophthalmol. 2017;65(12):1340–9.
6. Sheeladevi S, Lawrenson JG, Fielder AR, Suttle CM. Global prevalence of childhood cataract: a systematic review. Eye (Lond). 2016;30:1160–9.
7. Fakhoury O, Aziz A, Matonti F, Benso C, Belahda K, Denis D, et al. Epidemiologic and etiological characteristics of congenital cataract: study of 59 cases over 10 years. J Fr Ophtalmol. 2015;38:295–300.
8. Yi J, Yun J, Li ZK, Xu CT, Pan BR. Epidemiology and molecular genetics of congenital cataracts. Int J Ophthalmol. 2011;4(4):422–32.
9. Hejtmancik JF, Kaiser-Kupfer MI, Piatigorsky J. Molecular biology and inherited disorders of the eye lens. In: 8th, editor. The metabolic and molecular basis of inherited disease. New York: McGraw Hill; 2001. p. 6033–62.
10. Lloyd IC, Goss-Sampson M, Jeffrey BG, Kriss A, Russell-Eggitt I, Taylor D. Neonatal cataract: aetiology, pathogenesis and management. Eye (Lond). 1992;6(Pt 2):184–96.

11. Jobling AI, Augusteyn RC. What causes steroid cataracts? A review of steroid-induced posterior subcapsular cataracts. Clin Exp Optom. 2002;85(2):61–75.
12. Devi RR, Yao W, Vijayalakshmi P, Sergeev YV, Sundaresan P, Hejtmancik JF. Crystallin gene mutations in Indian families with inherited pediatric cataract. Mol Vis. 2008;14:1157–70. PMID: 18587492; PMCID: PMC2435160
13. Hejtmancik JF. Congenital cataracts and their molecular genetics. Semin Cell Dev Biol. 2008;19:134–49.
14. Santana A, Waiswo M. The genetic and molecular basis of congenital cataract. Arq Bras Oftalmol. 2011;74:136–42.
15. Shiels A, Hejtmancik JF. Genetics of human cataract. Clin Genet. 2013;84(2):120–7. https://doi.org/10.1111/cge.12182.
16. Huang B, He W. Molecular characteristics of inherited congenital cataracts. Eur J Med Genet. 2010;53:347–57.
17. Reddy MA, Francis PJ, Berry V, Bhattacharya SS, Moore AT. Molecular genetic basis of inherited cataract and associated phenotypes. Surv Ophthalmol. 2004;49:300–15.
18. Burdon KP, McKay JD, Wirth MG, Russell-Eggit IM, Bhatti S, Ruddle JB, et al. The PITX3 gene in posterior polar congenital cataract in Australia. Mol Vis. 2006;12:367–71.
19. Bökenkamp A, Ludwig M. The oculocerebrorenal syndrome of Lowe: an update. Pediatr Nephrol. 2016;31:2201–12.
20. Atik SU, Gürsoy S, Koçkar T, Önal H, Adal SE. Clinical, molecular, and genetic evaluation of galactosemia in Turkish children. Turk Pediatri Ars. 2016;51:204–9.
21. American Academy of Ophthalmology. Chapter 23: Childhood cataract and other pediatric lens disorders. In: Basic and clinical sciences course. Pediatric ophthalmology and strabismus 2015-2016. San Francisco, CA: American Academy of Ophthalmology; 2015. p. 291–308.
22. Tian Q, Li Y, Kousar R, et al. A novel NHS mutation causes Nance-Horan Syndrome in a Chinese family. BMC Med Genet. 2017;18(1):2. https://doi.org/10.1186/s12881-016-0360-9.
23. Ippel PF, Wittebol-post D, Van Nesselrooij BPM, Bijlsma JB. Sutural cataract, retinitis pigmentosa, microcephaly and psychomotor retardation a new autosomal recessive disorder? Ophthalmic Genet. 1994;15(3–4):121–7. https://doi.org/10.3109/13816819409057838.
24. Taylor D. Neonatal cataract: aetiology, pathogenesis and management. Eye. 1992;6:184–96.
25. Donaldson PJ. A link between maternal malnutrition and depletion of glutathione in the developing lens: a possible explanation for idiopathic childhood cataract? Clin Exp Optom. 2013;96:523–8.
26. Eckstein M, Vijayalakshmi P, Killedar M, Gilbert C, Foster A. Aetiology of childhood cataract in south India. Br J Ophthalmol. 1996;80:628–32.
27. Kohn A. The differential diagnosis of cataracts in infancy and childhood. Am J Dis Child. 1976;130:184–92.
28. Yenerel NM, Küçümen RB. Pregnancy and the eye. Turkish J Ophthalmol. 2015;45(5):213–9.
29. Russell-eggitt I, Lightman S. Intrauterine infection and the eye. Eye. 1992;6:205–10.
30. Wilson BME. Pediatric cataracts: overview. In: American Academy of Ophthalmology. p. 1–25; 2015.
31. Cibis A, Burde RM, Louis S. Herpes simplex virus-induced congenital cataracts. Arch Ophthal. 1971;85:220–3.
32. Cotlier E. Congenital varicella cataract. Am J Ophthalmol [Internet]. 1978;86(5):627–9. https://doi.org/10.1016/0002-9394(78)90180-0.
33. Mansoor N, Mansoor T, Ahmed M. Eye pathologies in neonates. Int J Ophthalmol. 2016;9(12):1832–8.
34. Raghu H, Subhan S, Jose RJ, Gangopadhyay N, Bhende J, Sharma S. Herpes Simplex Virus-1 – Associated congenital cataract. Am J Ophthalmol. 2004;138(2):313–4.
35. Vutova K, Peicheva Z, Popova A, Markova V, Mincheva N. Congenital toxoplasmosis: eye manifestations in infants and children. Ann Trop Paediatr. 2002:213–8.
36. Endres W, Shin YS. Cataract and metabolic disease. J Inher Metab Dis. 1990;13:509–16.
37. Trumler AA. Evaluation of pediatric cataracts and systemic disorders. Curr Opin Ophthalmol. 2011;22:365–79.

38. Kaya A. Preoperative usage of ultrasound biomicroscopy in pediatric cataract. Arq Bras Oftalmol. 2016;79:62.
39. Kaur S, Yangzes S, Ram J. Unilateral congenital cataract. J Pediatr Ophthalmol Strabismus. 2019;56:60–1.
40. Spencer T, Mamalis N. The pathology of cataracts. In: Steinert R, editor. Cataract surgery. 3rd ed. Saunders Elsevier: Irvine, CA; 2010. p. 4–6.
41. Haargaard B. Down's syndrome and early cataract. Br J Ophthalmol. 2006;90(8):1024–7. https://doi.org/10.1136/bjo.2006.090639.
42. Koole FD, Velzeboer CMJ, Van Der Harten JJ. Ocular abnormalities in Patau syndrome (chromosome 13 trisomy syndrome). Ophthal Paediatr Genet. 1990;11(1):15–21. https://doi.org/10.3109/13816819009012944.
43. Cogan DG, Kuwabara T. Ocular pathology of the 13-15 trisomy syndrome. Archiv Ophthalmol. 1964;72(2):246–53. https://doi.org/10.1001/archopht.1964.00970020246021.
44. Pe'er J, Braun JT. Ocular pathology in trisomy 18 (Edwards' Syndrome). Ophthalmologica. 1986;192(3):176–8. https://doi.org/10.1159/000309637.
45. Mirmohammadsadeghi A, Akbari MR, Malekpoor A. Ocular manifestations in Edward's syndrome, a case report and literature review. J Curr Ophthalmol. 2017;29(4):329–31. https://doi.org/10.1016/j.joco.2017.06.005.
46. Denniston A, Butler L. Ophthalmic features of Turner's syndrome. Eye (Lond). 2004;18:680–4. https://doi.org/10.1038/sj.eye.6701323.
47. Lessell S, Forbes AP. Eye signs in Turner's syndrome. Archiv Ophthalmol. 1966;76(2):211–3. https://doi.org/10.1001/archopht.1966.03850010213011.
48. Gillespie RL, Sullivan JO, Ashworth J, Bhaskar S, Williams S, Biswas S, et al. Personalized diagnosis and management of congenital cataract by next-generation sequencing. Ophthalmology [Internet]. 2014;121(11):2124–37.e2. https://doi.org/10.1016/j.ophtha.2014.06.006.
49. Pichi F, Lembo A, Serafino M, Nucci P. Genetics of congenital cataract. Pediatr Cataract. 2016;57:1–14.
50. Francis PJ, Berry V, Bhattacharya SS, Moore AT. The genetics of childhood cataract. J Med Genet. 2000;37:481–8.
51. Gogate P, Sahasrabudhe M, Shah M, Patil S, Kulkarni A. Causes, epidemiology, and long-term outcome of traumatic cataracts in children in rural India. Indian J Ophthalmol. 2012;60(5):481–6.
52. Spencer T, Mamalis N. The pathology of cataracts. In: Steinert R, editor. Cataract surgery. 3rd ed. Saunders Elsevier: Irvine, CA; 2010. p. 3–10.
53. William Z. The pathogenesis of vossius ring cataract. Am J Ophthalmol. 1924;79:676–7.
54. Alekseev BN, Sibai SA. Opredelenie termina "oslozhnennye katarakty" [Definition of the term "complicated cataracts"]. Vestn Oftalmol. 1996;112(4):26–7.
55. Ganesh SK, Bala A, Biswas J, Ahmed AS, Kempen JH. Pattern of pediatric uveitis seen at a tertiary referral center from India. Ocul Immunol Inflamm. 2016;24:402–9.
56. Blum-Hareuveni T, Seguin-Greenstein S, Kramer M, Hareuveni G, Sharon Y, Friling R, et al. Risk factors for the development of cataract in children with uveitis. Am J Ophthalmol. 2017;177:139–43.
57. Lambert S, Drack A. Infantile cataracts. Surv Ophthalmol. 1996;40(6):427–58.
58. Henk JM, Whitelocke RAF, Warrington AP, Bessell EM. Radiation dose to the lens and cataract formation. Int J Radiat Oncol Biol Phys. 1993;25:815–20.

3 Preoperative Evaluation of Pediatric Cataract

Sudarshan Khokhar, Chirakshi Dhull, and Amber Amar Bhayana

3.1 Introduction

There are no substitutes to a thorough history and careful clinical examination while planning for any surgery and pediatric cataract is no different. Preoperative evaluation should be performed keeping the differential diagnoses in mind. Questions like the cause of the cataract, whether to operate, when to operate and how to operate should be answered by preoperative examination. Performing biometry and deciding the particulars of the intraocular lens implant including the post-operative target refraction are all equally challenging but essential prerequisites. With numerous uncertainties, a good preoperative planning is the key to successful management of pediatric cataract.

3.2 History

A child with cataract is usually brought by parents who notice leukocoria, strabismus, abnormal ocular movements or delayed visual milestones or if the poor vision has been pointed out by teachers in school. The reader must be aware of the differential diagnoses of similar presentation (Table 3.1). An older one may subjectively report diminished vision or glare depending on the morphology of the cataract.

In cases of trauma, the history is usually obvious. Details about the mechanism and severity will point towards an open or a closed globe injury. In an open globe a

S. Khokhar (✉) · A. A. Bhayana
Dr Rajendra Prasad Centre for Ophthalmic Sciences, All India Institute of Medical Sciences (AIIMS), New Delhi, India

C. Dhull
Eye Q Hospital, Gurugram, India

S. Agrawal (ed.), *Pediatric Cataract*,
https://doi.org/10.1007/978-981-16-1736-2_3

Table 3.1 Differential diagnosis in a child with leukocoria

Opacity anterior to lens
• Peters anomaly
• Corneal opacity
Lenticular opacity
• Isolated cataract
• Complicated cataract
Opacity posterior to lens
• Retinoblastoma
• Retinopathy of prematurity
• Retinal detachment
• Persistent fetal vasculature
• Vitreous haemorrhage
• Coats disease
• Toxocariasis

primary repair becomes essential. A rupture of the anterior or posterior lens capsule may alter the surgical plan as discussed later. In closed globe injury subluxation of lens, angle recession, sphincter or retinal tears are possible. Even in absence of an obvious history of trauma, signs of trauma must be actively looked for while evaluating unilateral pediatric cataracts.

Siblings and parents should always be screened in cases of non-traumatic congenital or developmental cataracts and pedigree chart for at least three generations documented. Genetic workup is warranted in presence of positive family history. Even in sporadic cases, genetic mutations might be involved most common of which are five nucleotide variations CRYBA4:p.Y67N, CRYBB1:p.D85N, CRYBB1:p.E75K, CRYBB1:p.E155K, and GJA3:p.M1V [1].

Other positive systemic histories may point towards a syndromic disorder. A thumb rule to keep in mind is that in cases of unilateral cataracts suspect something wrong in the eye itself, whereas in cases of bilateral cataracts some systemic or genetic disorder might be the culprit. It should also be remembered that many seemingly unilateral cataracts are actually asymmetrically bilateral. It would be useful here to go through the etiology of cataract in children discussed in detail in the previous chapter and summarised in Table 3.2 [2].

Mothers should be inquired about infections or exanthematous fever episodes during their antenatal period as 1st-trimester rubella infection is a common cause of congenital cataracts in developing nations. History and details of any drug use during the antenatal period must also be elicited. A false negative history for rubella infection due to mild illness during pregnancy or a recall bias may be misleading [3]. These children require a detailed systemic evaluation to rule out other systemic involvements (Table 3.3). Perinatal history regarding gestational age at delivery, mode of delivery, delayed cry should also be documented. In older children, treatment history including oral, topical ophthalmic and topical dermatological medications especially steroids, should be documented to rule out drug-induced cataracts.

Table 3.2 Etiology of cataract in children

Bilateral cataracts	**Unilateral cataracts**
Idiopathic	Idiopathic
Hereditary cataracts (autosomal dominant)	Ocular anomalies—persistent fetal vasculature, anterior segment dysgenesis, posterior lenticonus, posterior pole tumours
Chromosomal, metabolic and systemic diseases—Down syndrome, Lowe syndrome, galactosemia, Marfan syndrome, trisomy 13–15, hypoglycaemia, Alport syndrome, myotonic dystrophy, Fabry disease, hypoparathyroidism	Traumatic
Maternal infection—rubella, cytomegalovirus, varicella, syphilis, toxoplasmosis	Maternal infection—rubella
Ocular anomalies—aniridia, anterior segment dysgenesis	Asymmetric bilateral cataract
Corticosteroid induced	Secondary retinal detachment, uveitis

Table 3.3 Suggested workup for an infant with suspected Rubella syndrome [4]

Maternal history	Exanthematous fever during antenatal period
	Lack of history for vaccination against Rubella
Common clinical features in child	Microphthalmos
	Iris atrophy, iritis, iris hypoplasia
	Posterior synechiae
	Congenital cataract (nuclear cataract)
	Pigmentary retinopathy
Investigations	IgM Antibody
	Persisting infant rubella antibody titres (IgG)
	Polymerase chain reaction virus detection (blood/saliva)
	Cardiology opinion and echocardiography to rule out cardiac anomalies
	Brainstem evoked response audiometry to rule out sensorineural hearing loss

Presence of cataract at birth implies congenital, whereas occurrence between infancy and adolescence implies developmental onset. Delayed presentation often makes the identification of onset confusing but the typical morphology as detailed in the next section may be helpful in confirmation (e.g. central fetal nuclear, polar, sutural cataracts are congenital and zonular cataract involving infantile nucleus is developmental). When congenital onset cannot be ascertained the cataract should be labelled as developmental.

3.3 Examination

Babies who have not yet developed neck holding can be examined in mother's lap. Those with neck holding are most comfortable in shoulder hold as shown in Fig. 3.1 [5]. This position increases the area of contact with the mother and the child is at ease. Children older than 3 to 4 years can be assessed on slit lamp. It is logical to perform tests like visual acuity assessment, red reflex test/dynamic retinoscopy, pupillary reaction and assessment of ocular movements, which do not require touching the child before proceeding with the part of the examination likely to make the child uncooperative like slit lamp or fundus examination. To enhance cooperation, rewarding the child in between tests with a sweet or a small toy is a successful trick used by many pediatric ophthalmologists.

3.3.1 Vision Assessment in Children

The most basic form of indirect vision assessment in the absence of nystagmus or searching eye movements is the binocular fixation preference (BFP). For this, the child is made to fixate on an accommodative target (or a dimly lit torchlight) at 40 cm. The fixing eye (or either eye if there is no obvious deviation) is occluded and the other eye is forced to take up fixation. If fixation is taken up readily and maintained even after removal of the cover the fixation pattern is termed as central,

Fig. 3.1 Shoulder hold position to examine the child

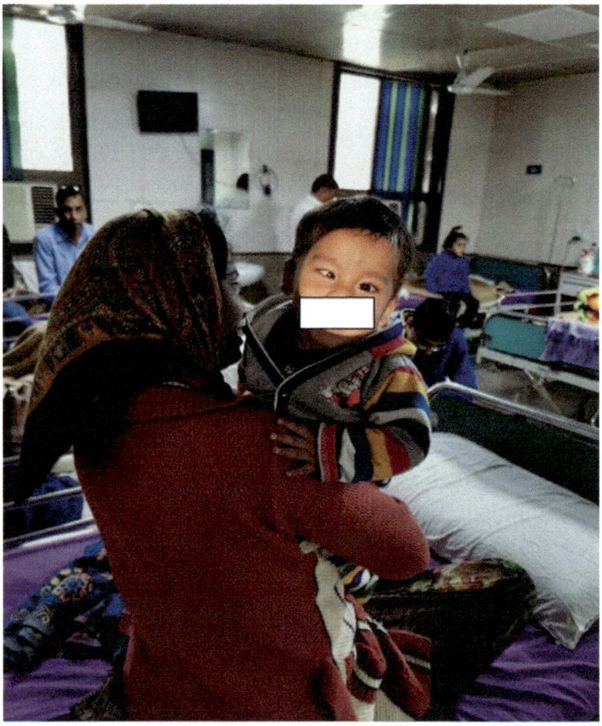

steady and maintained (CSM) [6]. If the fixation immediately shifts to the other eye on removal of the occluder the fixation is central, steady and unmaintained (CSUM). Similarly, if on occlusion of the fixing eye, the fixation in the other eye is central but wandering, the pattern is termed central, unsteady and unmaintained (CUSUM). If the eye does not take up fixation at all, it is termed as uncentral, unsteady and unmaintained (UCUSUM). BFP is indicative of an interocular difference in visual acuity, ranging from no difference in presence of CSM fixation in both eyes to 0.71 ± 48 (LogMAR) in presence of UCUSUM fixation in one eye [7]. Presence of nystagmus or searching eye movements indicates poor vision in both eyes.

For pre-verbal children, the following tests can be used: (1) Catford drum test makes use of oscillating dots of different sizes and visual acuity can be assessed by the smallest dot provoking pendular eye movements [8], (2) Teller acuity cards (Fig. 3.2) are based on preferential looking where the child prefers to look at gratings of alternating black and white stripes of maximum detectable frequency rather than a plain background, (3) Visual evoked response detects potential generated in the cerebral cortex in response to light stimulation and (4) Pupillary response is another indirect method to detect vision where an equal and brisk response grossly suggests normal visual pathway.

For pre-school children (about 2 years of age) following can be used: (1) Cardiff acuity cards (Fig. 3.3) based on the principle of vanishing optotypes where pictures are drawn of the same size but are drawn with black lines with white space of varying width so that they disappear at a particular distance, (2) Boeck candy test, where the child is offered candies of different sizes; smallest detectable candy being a measure of visual acuity, (3) Worth's ivory ball test, where balls of different sizes are rolled across the floor; the smallest ball, which the child can retrieve is a measure of visual acuity, (4) Similarly, in Sheridan's ball test, fixation on rolling balls is assessed and (5) In STYCAR, the child is asked to name the shown toy or pick up its miniature form from the stock.

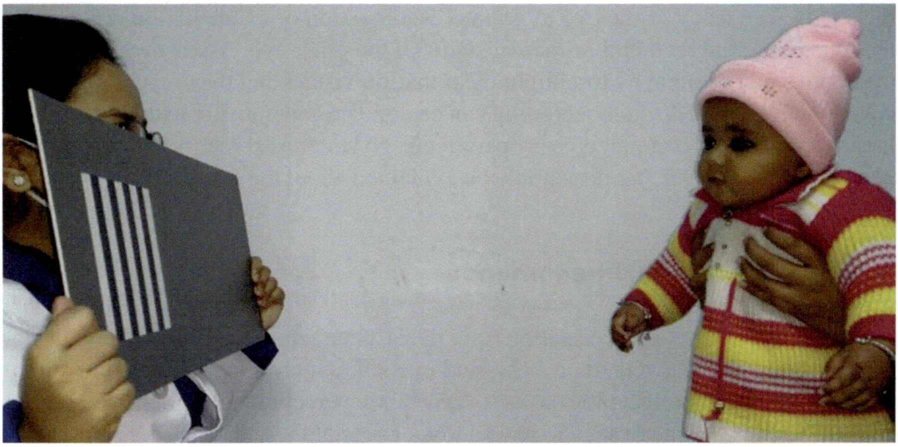

Fig. 3.2 Vision assessment with Teller Acuity Cards (Stereo Optical Co, Chicago, IL)

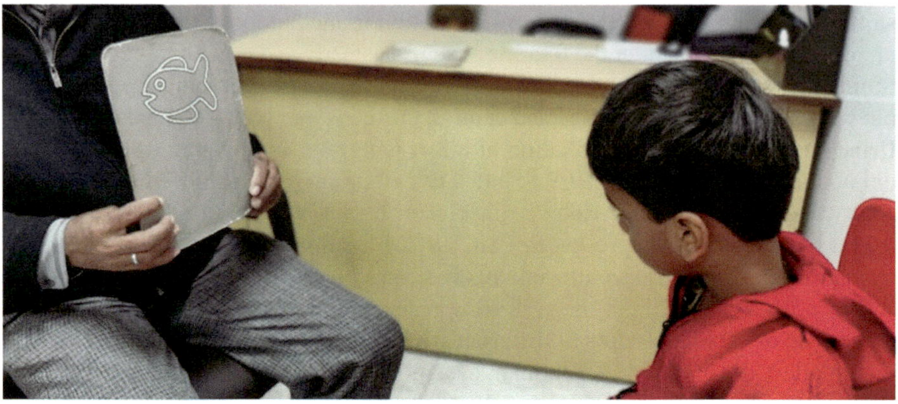

Fig. 3.3 Vision assessment using Cardiff acuity cards

For ages more than 5 years Tumbling E, Landolt C charts can be used and Snellen thereafter [9].

A binocular vision better than uniocular is due to binocular summation and representative of a certain level of binocularity [10].

Table 3.4 summarises different methods to assess visual acuity in different ages.

3.3.2 Ocular Movements

Children with visually significant cataracts with onset before 3 months of age are likely to have nystagmus because the media opacity prevents the development of fixation reflex [11]. This nystagmus is likely to persist even after media clarity is restored. Post-treatment best-corrected vision in such patients is seldom better than 20/100. Similarly, wandering eye movements and ocular deviation are generally associated with poor prognosis. Presence of strabismus indicates chronicity in cataracts [11]. Tendency of the eye to go into esodeviation or exodeviation depends on the tone of medial recti and refractive status of the other eye. Assessment of squint/nystagmus can be done by torchlight examination visualising the corneal reflex and cover uncover tests. A video recording can be done pre-operatively to document ocular movements and compared post-operatively. Nystagmus sometimes may improve post-surgery, however, parents should be explained about the guarded prognosis [9].

3.3.3 Oculo-digital Phenomenon

Infants with gross visual deprivation as in dense cataracts are seen to poke their fingers in the groove between their brow and eyeball, which is hypothesised to stimulate their retinal photoreceptors so as to have some perception of light in the form of flashes. Such children are seen to have a loss of orbital fat with deep-set globes with poor fixation and wandering eye movements, all indicating poor visual prognosis (Fig. 3.4) [12].

Table 3.4 Methods to assess visual acuity at different ages

Preverbal
• Pupillary reflexes
• Visual evoked response
• Optokinetic nystagmus
• Teller acuity
• Pattern of fixation
1–2 years
• Worth's ivory ball test
• Boeck candy test
• Screening test for the young children and retards
• Cardiff acuity test
2–3 years
• Miniature toy test
• Coin test
• LEA Symbols
3–5 years
• Allen picture card
• Lippman's HOTV test, letter test
>5 years
• Tumbling E
• Landolt broken ring
• Snellen chart
• LogMAR chart

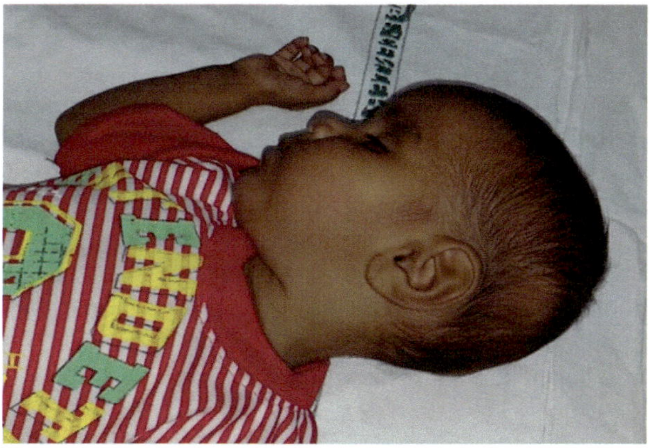

Fig. 3.4 Child with orbital fat atrophy secondary to excessive-digital phenomenon

3.3.4 Pupils

Pupils should be examined before dilation. Size, shape, interocular symmetry should be documented. Signs of blunt trauma like sphincter tears, iridodialysis should be looked for in respective cases. Direct and consensual responses should be checked and any relative afferent pupillary defect should be carefully looked for; if present indicates neuronal damage.

3.3.5 Red Reflex Test

Distant direct ophthalmoscopy enables assessment of the red glow of the eye, which is sensitive for detection of visual axis opacities, refractive errors, anisometropia and strabismus (Bruckner test) (Fig. 3.5). It is a handy and useful test that can be used even in uncooperative children [13–16]. It may be done after mydriasis or prior to it in a dark room. Based on the same test, photography with flashlight may be used for screening several amblyogenic conditions in children [17].

3.3.6 Anterior Segment Examination

Evaluation of anterior segment can be done on slit lamp biomicroscope (if the child allows) or else with torchlight. Any doubt should warrant an examination under sedation or anaesthesia. Lid and adnexa should be thoroughly checked for any discharge, nasolacrimal duct obstruction, blepharitis or any other foci of active infections. Corneal opacities, abnormalities of anterior chamber, iris and pupil should be documented. Signs of inflammation like posterior synechiae or cells in anterior chamber along with band-shaped keratopathy are suggestive of complicated cataract and are often found associated with juvenile idiopathic arthritis (JIA) [18]. Microphthalmos and typical colobomas are also frequently associated with congenital/developmental cataracts. Presence of small corneal opacity or an iris hole could be a tell-tale sign of penetrating ocular trauma in unilateral cases.

3.3.7 Lens Examination

A thorough examination of the cataractous lens can not only aid morphological classification but can also suggest possible etiology (Tables 3.2 and 3.5; Figs. 3.6, 3.7, 3.8, 3.9, and 3.10) [2, 19].

Bilateral zonular cataracts are most commonly sporadic/developmental whereas unilateral cataracts maybe post-trauma or iatrogenic (such as after trabeculectomy and retinopathy of prematurity surgeries); morphologically presenting most commonly as posterior subcapsular (PSC) variants [20, 21]. Unilateral presentation may also be due to asymmetry of bilateral cataracts as mentioned earlier. A good slit lamp

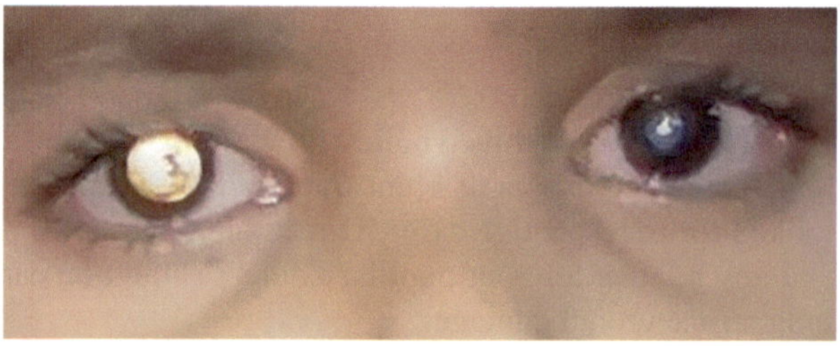

Fig. 3.5 Bruckner test showing a cataractous lens in left eye

Table 3.5 Morphological classification of pediatric cataract based on location of the opacity

Whole lens	Central	Anterior	Posterior	Miscellaneous
Total	Lamellar/ zonular	Anterior polar (a) Dot like (b) Plaque like (c) Pyramidal	Posterior polar	Oil droplet
Congenital morgagnian	Nuclear	Anterior subcapsular	Posterior subcapsular	Wedge shaped
Membranous/ partially absorbed	Central pulverulent	Anterior lenticonus	Posterior lenticonus	Coralliform
	Ant egg			Floriform
	Cerulean cataract			Dandelion like
	Cortical			Starry sky cataract
	Sutural			Stud button
				Reduplicated cataract
				Linear opacities
				Crystalline
				Nodular
				Stem of cactus
				Barbed fence-like cataract

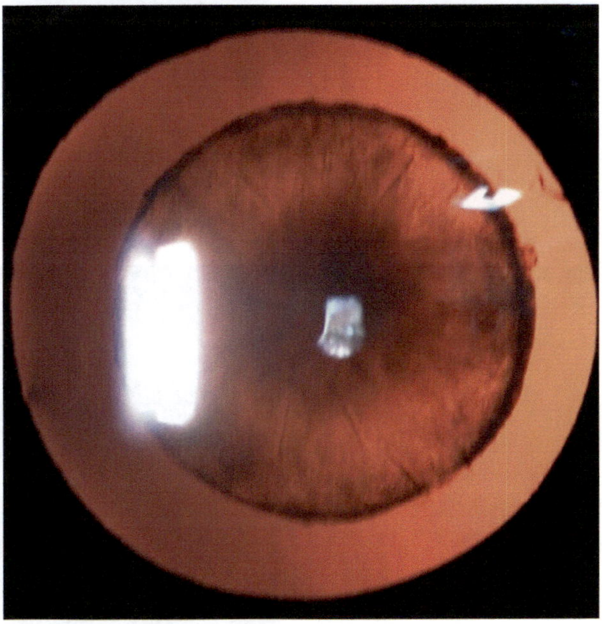

Fig. 3.6 Zonular cataract

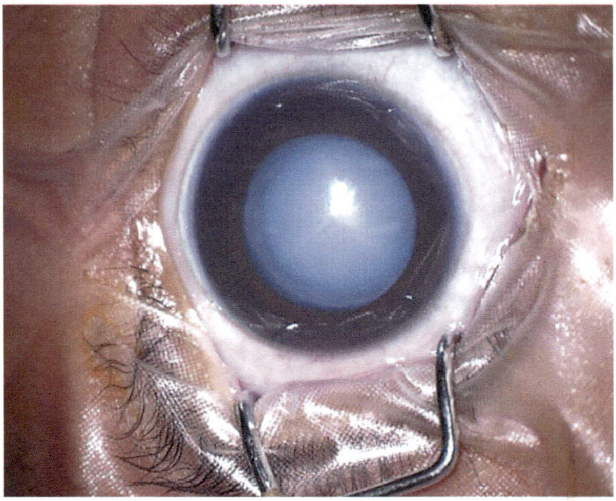

Fig. 3.7 Total white cataract

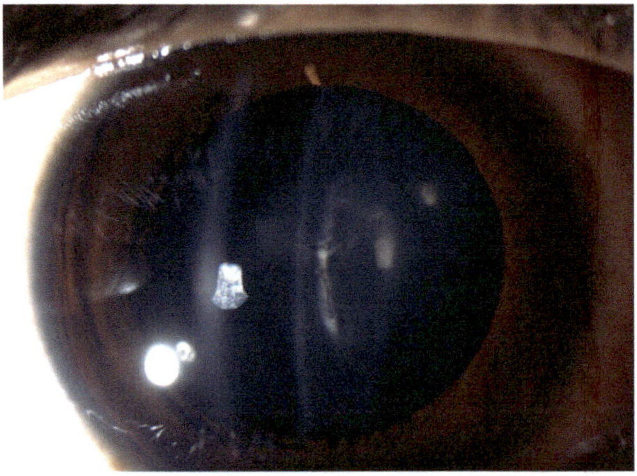

Fig. 3.8 Sutural cataract

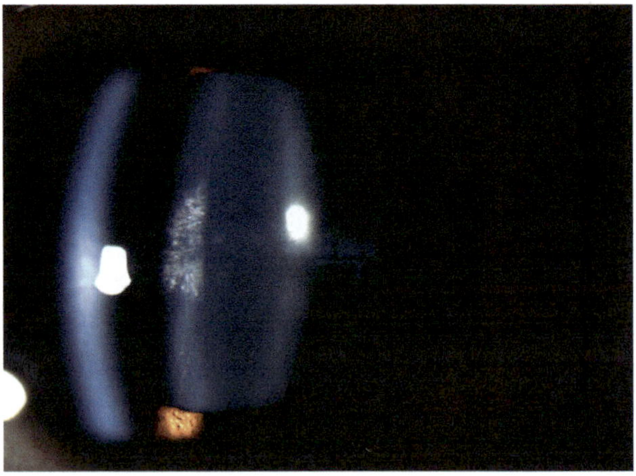

Fig. 3.9 Anterior capsular cataract

biomicroscopic assessment of apparently normal eye is essential in unilateral cases. Traumatic cataracts can be post closed globe injuries or more commonly post open globe injuries (Fig. 3.11) [22]. A rosette-shaped cataract is often associated with blunt trauma whereas membranous or total may be found associated with penetrating trauma [23, 24]. Total cataracts may also be present in chromosomal anomalies or metabolic disorders. Bilateral PSCs may indicate chronic steroid intake. In addition to nuclear lenticular opacity, poorly dilating pupils with partially absorbed cataract and posterior synechiae in a microphthalmic eye may indicate rubella. Flat anterior curvature of the lens may indicate posterior capsular rupture which may be picked up on slit lamp biomicroscopy as "fish-tail" sign or on ultrasound B-scan and ultrasound biomicroscopy. Persistent pupillary membrane might be a coexisting finding which is indicative of remnant fetal lenticular vasculature found attached at the collarette.

Cataracts that cause significant obstruction to fundal glow and opacities greater than 3 mm in the visual axis need surgical intervention. Lenticular opacities in the periphery not causing hindrance to visual axis can simply be observed over time (Fig. 3.12).

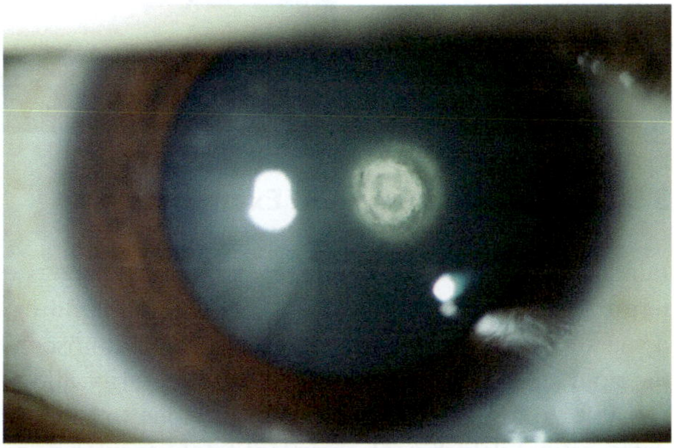

Fig. 3.10 Posterior polar cataract

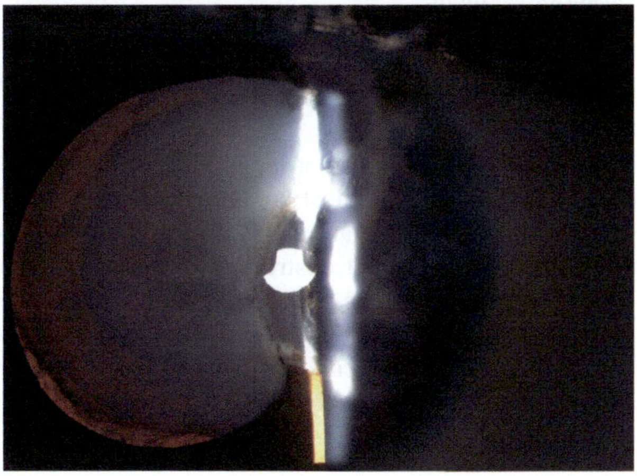

Fig. 3.11 Traumatic cataract following corneal perforation

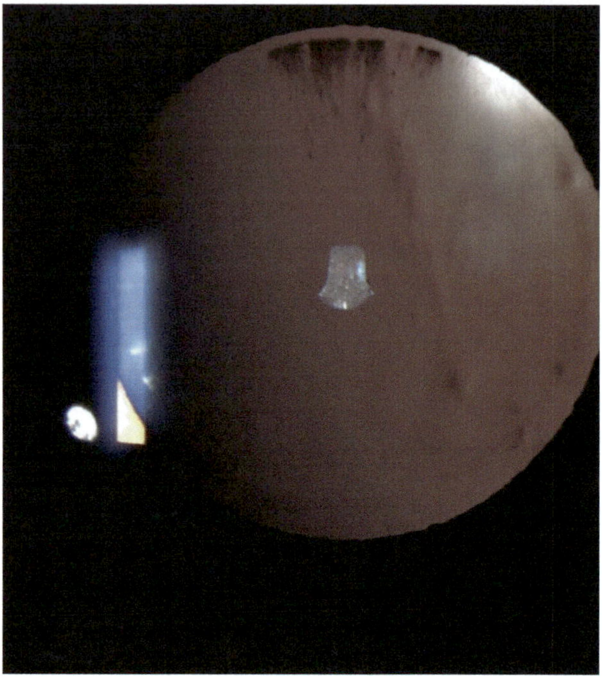

Fig. 3.12 Visually insignificant cataract

3.3.8 Posterior Segment Examination

Fundus examination with indirect ophthalmoscope is essential to rule out any posterior segment anomaly that may prevent the child from gaining vision even after a successful cataract surgery. Indirect ophthalmoscopy with scleral indentation is the gold standard if the child and media clarity allow. If view of the retina is not possible, ultrasound B-scan should be done to rule out vitreous haemorrhage/exudates, retinal detachment persistent fetal vasculature or any intraocular mass in the posterior segment.

3.4 Syndromic Associations

These have been discussed at length in the previous chapter. Down syndrome (trisomy 21) is one of the most common chromosomal abnormalities having a wide range of ocular manifestations like mongoloid slant, esotropia, nystagmus, refractive errors, lacrimal duct obstruction, Brushfield's spots on iris and keratoconus. Prevalence of cataracts in such patients varies from 4 to 37% [25]. Lowe syndrome (oculocerebrorenal disorder) causes congenital cataracts, lenticonus (Fig. 3.13), mental retardation and renal dysfunction [26]. Features of congenital rubella syndrome include microcephaly, sensorineural deafness, patent ductus arteriosus and ocular involvements some of which include membranous cataract with poorly

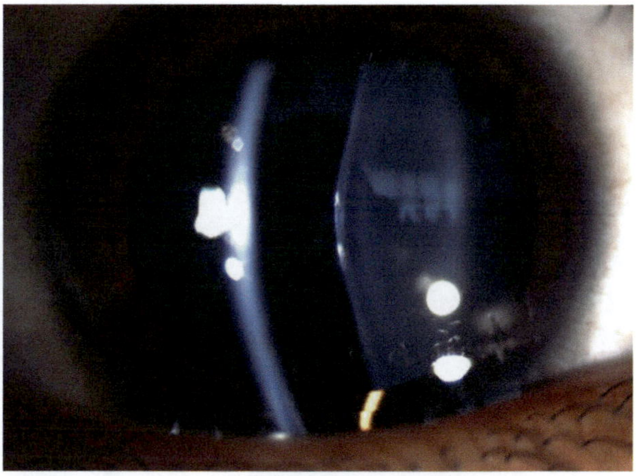

Fig. 3.13 Anterior lenticonus

dilating pupil, posterior synechiae, microphthalmos and salt and pepper retinopathy [27]. IgM and IgG titres should be sent for if suspected. Cataract in an infant with hepatomegaly, failure to thrive and jaundice should raise suspicion of galactosemia and be investigated accordingly [28].

3.5 Investigations

Majority of the cataracts are idiopathic and do not require extensive investigations. However, labelling the cataract as idiopathic should only be done after excluding the obvious causes.

1. Etiology specific investigations should be done only after a detailed clinical examination with a possible diagnosis in mind. For example, a child having cataract with hepatomegaly should be investigated for galactosemia (urinary reducing substance, galactokinase and galactose 1-phosphate uridyl transferase enzyme levels). For suspected infectious etiology like rubella, immunoglobulin levels are warranted along with polymerase chain reaction targeted towards other viruses in TORCH spectrum. Echocardiography is required to rule out cardiac anomalies in rubella which might also be present in cases of Marfan syndrome. The common anomalies encountered are atrial septal defects, patent ductus arteriosus and aortic root dilatation. In suspected cases of hypothyroidism, serum calcium and phosphorus levels need to be looked into. In patients with juvenile idiopathic arthritis-related cataracts, a detailed rheumatology workup is warranted. Genetic testing is warranted in cases of hereditary cataracts.
2. Imaging:
   (a) Ultrasound (USG) B-scan is warranted in cases of significant media opacities where fundus evaluation on indirect ophthalmoscopy is not possible as in cases with total cataracts or poorly dilating pupils to get an impression of the

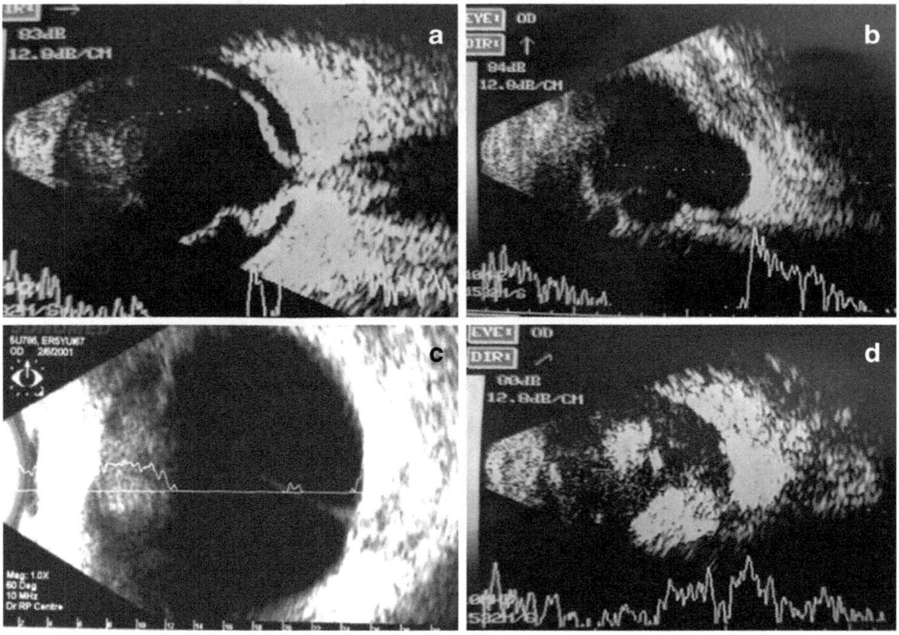

Fig. 3.14 Posterior segment ultrasound B-scan images showing (**a**) Retinal detachment, (**b**) Fundal coloboma, (**c**) Persistent fetal vasculature, (**d**) Retinoblastoma (Courtesy: Khokhar S, Dhull C, Atlas of Pediatric Cataract, Springer Ltd.)

posterior segment. Retinal detachments (Fig. 3.14a), fundal colobomas (Fig. 3.14b), persistent fetal vasculature (PFV) (Fig. 3.14c) or any mass in posterior segment like retinoblastoma or melanoma (Fig. 3.14d) can be easily picked up [29]. It is also useful in very small children who are uncooperative for examination. A vector modality over B-scan (A on B scan) is used to take ocular measurements mainly of the axial length or can be used to measure intraocular dimension of any mass.

(b) Ultrasound biomicroscopy (UBM) uses ultrasound frequencies in the range of 50–100 MHz, unlike the conventional B-scan which utilises about 10 MHz [30]. UBM enables high-resolution examination of the anterior segment (Fig. 3.15). It has special utility in identifying posterior polar cataract, pre-existing posterior capsular defect and anterior PFV [31]. In presence of trauma, it may additionally identify cyclodialysis, subluxation of crystalline lens and presence of a foreign body [32]. Its utility is enhanced in the presence of media opacity. UBM is also very useful for post-operative complications like visual axis opacification (VAO) and glaucoma to identify the altered anatomy and to plan management.

(c) Magnetic Resonance Imaging or Colour Doppler may be indicated to confirm PFV when the clinical suspicion is high and findings on USG inconclusive.

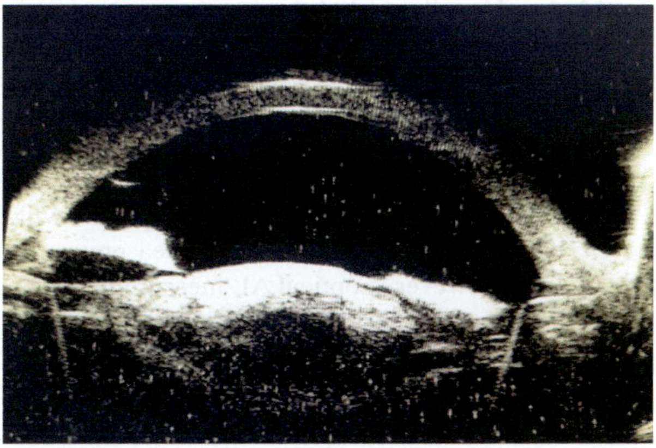

Fig. 3.15 Ultrasound Biomicroscopy (UBM) image of a 16 month old child, showing cataract involving anterior part of the lens with a deep anterior chamber on right side

   (d) X-ray skull (PA and lateral views) and/or computed tomography are done in trauma for bone injury and to localise an intraocular foreign body.
3. Electrophysiological tests like electroretinography and visual evoked potential, may selectively be performed for prognostication by assessment of retinal function and detection of stimulus deprivation amblyopia [33].
4. General anaesthesia (GA) workup warrants complete blood counts with electrolytes as routine for any surgery. In infants, haemoglobin, bleeding, clotting times and urine microscopy may be required. Targeted investigations like chest X-ray, ECG and echocardiogram should be done in patients with diagnosed specific systemic disorders for pre-anaesthetic fitness. A consultation from the respective specialist should be sought. A child with seizure will require anti-epileptic dose modification for the peri-operative and intraoperative period by the treating neurologist. Final clearance is given by the anaesthetist after complete systemic evaluation. Simultaneous bilateral cataract surgery may be a feasible option in patients with increased risk for repeated GA.

3.6 Surgical Planning

It involves planning issues related to biometry, choice and power of IOL, surgical preparation and procedure of choice. The details of planning are discussed under the following heads:

1. Biometry
   (a) Keratometry can be done using autorefractor-keratometer or portable handheld keratometer under anaesthesia. Partial coherence interferometry utilising machines (like IOL Master, Carl Zeiss Meditec; and LenStar, Haag Streit) may be used wherever possible. The keratometry at birth is about 52 D which reduces rapidly in the first 6 months and then slowly to reach an adult value of about 44 D at 2–3 years of age [34]. Keratometry should be performed without speculum [35].

(b) Axial length (AL) of the eye can be measured by ultrasound A-scan. When the probe is placed perpendicular to the eyeball parallel to its axis, the retina is picked up as a sharply rising echo spike. This is the contact method in which the probe may indent the cornea and may give falsely lower value of AL [36]. To overcome this error, a useful tip is to use for calculations the AL reading with the maximum anterior chamber depth [37]. A better method is the immersion technique in which a coupling fluid is used between the probe and the cornea preventing errors due to indentation. Ideal however is optical AL measurement using partial coherence interferometry (as using IOL Master, Carl Zeiss) which is a non-contact, observer-independent, reproducible and more accurate method (Fig. 3.16). But this can be used only for cooperative children over 4 year old. A-scan under anaesthesia (using immersion technique) just prior to surgery is the best option in smaller children. It should be kept in mind that an error of 1 mm in AL measurement causes an error of about 2.5 D in IOL power calculation. The A-scan used should have an oscilloscope screen for confirming the echo spikes from the retina and ensuring true axial measurement. Instruments that only provide the numerical reading of the AL should be avoided.

Determining the target post-operative refraction and selecting the appropriate IOL calculation formula are challenging as pediatric eyes grow until their pre-programmed adult sizes are reached. This destined adult size is affected by a number of variables like the age of onset of cataract (congenital/developmental), age of surgery, status of the other eye and presence of IOL in the eye. The calculation errors are largest with AL lesser than 20 mm and age of children below 36 months [38]. The preferred IOL formulae in children are SRK/T and Holladay 2 as they have been shown to have least predictive error [39].

It is desirable to target moderate hypermetropia in the immediate post-operative period in anticipation of the eye to gradually grow into emmetropia.

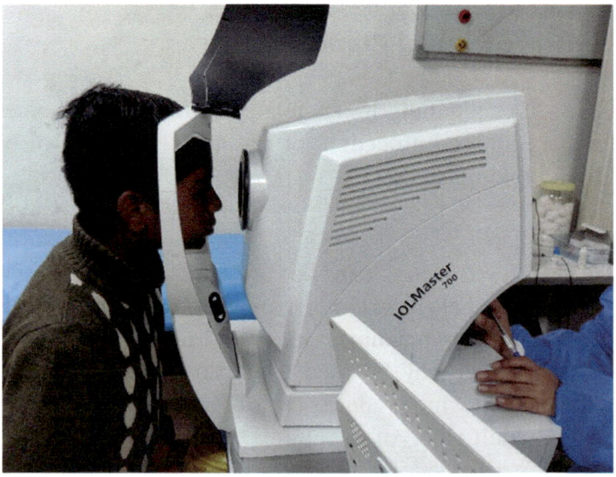

Fig. 3.16 Older children are cooperative for optical biometry

For this, the power of the IOL implanted is reduced by a predetermined percentage (under corrected) from the calculated IOL power. However, it should be understood that if significant undercorrection of IOL power is done there is a risk of hypermetropic amblyopia and if post-operative emmetropia is planned, every 1 mm growth in axial length will cause 3 dioptres of myopia as the child grows. Thus, a balance between the two has to be achieved. While there are several calculation nomograms the general principle is to do a lesser undercorrection (closer to emmetropia) in older children, unilateral cases, expected poor post-operative compliance and where parents are hypermetropic.

There are conflicting reports in literature regarding the desirable undercorrection from the calculated IOL power. Dahan et al. proposed a 20% reduction for children less than 2 years of age and 10% reduction for children between 2 and 8 years of age and emmetropic power thereafter [40]. On the basis of axial length he proposed 19 D for 21 mm, 21 D for 20 mm, 23 D for 19 mm, 24 D for 18 mm and 25 D for 17 mm. Enyedi et al. proposed age (years) + post of refractive error (dioptres) should be equal to 7 [41].

What we follow for our patients is 20% undercorrection for less than 6 months age, 15% for 6 months to 1 year, 10% for 1–2 years, 5% for 2–5 years and emmetropic power thereafter. Besides poor compliance to post-operative optical correction and occlusion, lesser undercorrection in Indian pediatric eyes is also justified by a study done by the authors in which the growth rate in Indian eyes was found to be less than the Western data [42]. We prefer not to put an implant if the AL is less than 17 mm or white to white corneal diameter is less than 9 mm [2]. Secondary IOL implantation can be planned later in these cases. These issues about IOLs have also been discussed in the next chapter.

2. Delayed sequential/simultaneous sequential bilateral surgery

   The main advantages of simultaneous bilateral cataract surgeries include medical benefits like single admission, undergoing anaesthesia only once; social benefits like requiring lesser time from caregivers and financial benefits with lesser surgical costs and lesser follow ups [43]. Risks include dreaded possibility of bilateral endophthalmitis and inability to evaluate refractive outcomes after first eye surgery, which can be later used to modify IOL power for the second eye [44]. To minimise the risk and maximise the benefits of both, we perform second eye surgery with a gap of 3 days or later. Simultaneous surgeries are done after detailed parental consent in infants who are at high risk for anaesthesia and where an intraocular implant is not planned.

3. Preoperative regimen of oral/topical medication

   Preoperatively the children are started on 0.5% moxifloxacin eye drops in both eyes for perioperative antibiotic coverage 2 days prior to surgery. Two percent homatropine hydrobromide is also instilled 1 day prior to surgery to ensure mydriasis. Infants and children with non-dilating pupils may require 1% atropine eye ointment twice daily for 3 days preoperatively.

4. Planning for additional procedures

   One of the commonest complications post pediatric cataract surgery is visual axis opacification (VAO), which occurs due to proliferation of remnant lens epithelial cells over the posterior capsule and/or vitreous scaffold. It occurs more commonly in younger children due to rapid proliferative capacity of lens epithelial cells in them. VAO is prevented or delayed by additional procedures like primary posterior capsulorhexis with or without limited anterior vitrectomy done in children below 6 years or those expected to be uncooperative for laser capsulotomy later. Size of the posterior capsular opening should be 4 to 4.5 mm about 1 mm smaller than anterior opening [2]. These procedures are discussed in detail in Chap. 5. Children who still develop VAO may require a second procedure like surgical capsulectomy for its timely management.
5. Options of IOLs

   With/without posterior rhexis, in the bag implantation of foldable hydrophobic acrylic white lenses with square edges is the preferred management of pediatric cataracts with good bag size. In cases of small bag size, complicated cases with extension of rhexis, inadvertent large posterior capsular opening, cases post-trauma with good sulcus support a multipiece lens can be implanted in the sulcus whose optic can be captured behind the posterior capsular opening to enhance its stability. Cases with subluxation greater than 8 clock hours that cannot be managed by capsular tension ring or Cionni bag fixation, are planned for scleral fixation of a multipiece lens provided the sclera is normal and there is no connective tissue disorder. Anterior chamber and iris claw lens are alternatives. The same options hold true for secondary IOL placement in cases left primarily aphakic. The IOL options in children and issues related to them are discussed in the next chapter.

3.7 Parent Counselling

Counselling is perhaps the most important step while planning any surgery. Parents/guardians need to be clearly explained in detail about the various issues. They must understand that even after a good surgery, post-operative visual gain may be poor due to amblyopia, and abnormality of the posterior segment whose assessment may not have been possible preoperatively. Parents have to be counselled regarding abnormal eye movements, long-term implications thereof and that the child will be dependent on spectacles life long for distance as well as near vision. Parents should be ready for long-term timely follow ups, use of spectacles and occlusion therapy for amblyopia management. All efforts must be taken to quench the queries of anxious parents to build a healthy rapport between the physician and the parents. A long and trustful association between doctors and parents is a necessary ingredient in management of pediatric cataract.

3.8 Summary

- Presenting features of pediatric cataracts include leukocoria, strabismus, abnormal ocular movements and delayed visual milestones.
- Differential diagnosis of leukocoria should be kept in mind to rule out causes other than cataract.
- Family members, especially siblings should always be screened.
- History of exanthematous fever during pregnancy may point towards congenital rubella infection.
- Bilateral cataracts have something abnormal in the body, unilateral cataracts have something abnormal in the eye.
- Small children can be examined in a mother's lap or shoulder hold.
- Vision assessment is the most elementary investigation that can be done using specialised tests depending on the age of child.
- Ocular movements, pupillary reaction and red reflex test are crucial parts of pediatric cataract assessment.
- Cataract morphology should be assessed on distant direct ophthalmoscopy as well as on slit lamp examination.
- Indirect ophthalmoscopy with scleral indentation is the gold standard for posterior segment evaluation wherever possible.
- Systemic investigations should be tailor cut and based on clinical clues.
- Ultrasound B-scan should be done in total media opacity.
- Prefer 20% undercorrection in IOL power for infants less than 6 months, 15% for 6 months to 1 year, 10% for 1–2 years, 5% for 2–5 years and emmetropic power thereafter.
- IOL should not be put in eyes with axial length lesser than 17 mm or white to white diameter lesser than 9 mm.

Multiple Choice Questions

1. Red reflex test helps us assess all *except*:
   (a) Refractive errors
   (b) Squint
   (c) Cataract
   (d) Glaucoma

   Answer: *d. Glaucoma.* Red reflex test or Bruckner test detects the asymmetry in red glow. Media opacities, ocular malalignment and refractive errors affect it whereas glaucoma does not.

2. Undercorrection percentage (%)in IOL power for infants less than 6 months with bilateral congenital cataract should be:
   (a) 20
   (b) 15

(c) 10
(d) 5

Answer: *a. 20%.* Undercorrection is recommended to compensate for the growth of eye later in life. Approximately 20% undercorrection is recommended for children up to 6 months of age with bilateral cataract. Lesser undercorrection is done for older children and those with unilateral cataract.

3. Which of the following is associated with lenticonus:
   (a) Down syndrome
   (b) Marfan syndrome
   (c) Alport syndrome
   (d) Ehlers Danlos syndrome

   Answer: c. *Alport syndrome*. Alport syndrome is associated with anterior lenticonus.

4. Fishtail and white dot sign are indicative of
   (a) Asteroid hyalosis
   (b) Synchysis scintillans
   (c) Posterior capsular rupture
   (d) Posterior polar cataract

   Answer: c. *Posterior capsular rupture.* The diagnostic signs of a pre-existing posterior capsule defect in children which can be seen preoperatively on slit lamp examination include a well-demarcated defect with thick margins, white spots in a cluster or a rough circle over the posterior capsule, and white dots in anterior vitreous that move with the degenerated vitreous such as a fishtail sign.

5. Best option for treatment for anisometropic amblyopia is:
   (a) Occlusion therapy
   (b) Glasses with occlusion
   (c) Contact lens with occlusion
   (d) Refractive lens exchange with occlusion

   Answer: c. *Contact lens with occlusion*. Glasses cause aniseikonia (asymmetrical size of images) in anisometropia which is minimised by contact lens. Occlusion of the better eye is the primary treatment of unilateral amblyopia.

6. Which of the following is not a differential diagnosis of congenital cataract:
   (a) Retinoblastoma
   (b) Persistent fetal vasculature syndrome
   (c) Coats disease
   (d) Typical iris coloboma

Answer: *d. Typical iris coloboma.* Typical iris coloboma presents as a defect in the iris inferonasally. The other three conditions cause opacity behind the lens which may present as white pupillary reflex.

References

1. Kumar M, Agarwal T, Kaur P, Kumar M, Khokhar S, Dada R. Molecular and structural analysis of genetic variations in congenital cataract. Mol Vis. 2013;19:2436–50.
2. Khokhar SK, Pillay G, Dhull C, Agarwal E, Mahabir M, Aggarwal P. Pediatric cataract. Indian J Ophthalmol. 2017;65:1340–9.
3. Eckstein M, Vijayalakshmi P, Killedar M, Gilbert C, Foster A. Aetiology of childhood cataract in south India. Br J Ophthalmol. 1996 Jul;80(7):628–32.
4. Lanzieri T, Redd S, Abernathy E, Icenogle J. Surveillance Manual | Congenital Rubella Syndrome | Vpds | Vaccines | CDC. [online] Cdc.gov. 2020. https://www.cdc.gov/vaccines/pubs/surv-manual/chpt15-crs.html
5. Khokhar SK, Dhull C. Atlas of pediatric cataract. Springer Nature Singapore; 2019. p. 128.
6. Wilson ME, Trivedi RH. Pediatric cataract surgery-techniques, complications and management. 2nd ed. Lipincott Williams and Wilkins, Wolters Kluwer. p. 34.
7. Kothari M, Bhaskare A, Mete D, Toshniwal S, Doshi P, Kaul S. Evaluation of central, steady, maintained fixation grading for predicting inter-eye visual acuity difference to diagnose and treat amblyopia in strabismic patients. Indian J Ophthalmol. 2009;57:281–4.
8. Sharma P. Strabismus simplified. 2nd ed. CBS publishers and distributors; 2016. p. 58.
9. Gole G. Visual acuity assessment in children. Clin Exp Ophthalmol. 1989;17:1–2.
10. Azen SP, Varma R, Preston-Martin S, Ying-Lai M, Globe D, Hahn S. Binocular visual acuity summation and inhibition in an ocular epidemiological study: the Los Angeles Latino eye study. Invest Ophthalmol Vis Sci. 2002;43:1742–8.
11. Rabiah PK, Smith SD, Awad AH, Al-garni A, Al-mesfer SA, Al-turkmani S, et al. Results of surgery for bilateral cataract associated with sensory nystagmus in children. Am J Ophthalmol. 2002;134:586–91.
12. Mansour AM, Reinecke RD. The pop eye phenomenon: an extreme form of the oculodigital phenomenon. J Clin Neuroophthalmol. 1985;5(4):281–2.
13. Tongue AC, Cibis GW. Bruckner test. Ophthalmology. 1981;88:1041–4.
14. Kothari MT. Can the Bruckner test be used as a rapid screening test to detect significant refractive errors in children? Indian J Ophthalmol. 2007;55:213–5.
15. Bhayana AA, Prasad P, Azad SV. Refractive errors and the red reflex – Bruckner test revisited. Indian J Ophthalmol. 2019;67:1381–2.
16. Bhayana AA. Response to comments on: using Brückner's test for gross keratometry screening. Indian J Ophthalmol. 2020;68:263.
17. Gupta R, Agrawal S, Srivastava RM, Singh V, Katiyar V. Smartphone photography for screening amblyogenic conditions in children. Indian J Ophthalmol. 2019;67:1560–3.
18. Clarke SL, Sen ES, Ramanan AV. Juvenile idiopathic arthritis-associated uveitis. Pediatr Rheumatol Online J. 2016;14(1):27.
19. Khokhar SK, Dhull C. Atlas of pediatric cataract. Springer Nature Singapore; 2019. p. 1.
20. Dada T, Bhartiya S, Baig NB. Cataract surgery in eyes with previous glaucoma surgery: pearls and pitfalls. J Curr Glaucoma Pract. 2013;7(3):99–105.
21. Chandra P, Khokhar S, Kumar A. Bilateral total cataract after laser treatment of aggressive posterior retinopathy of prematurity. Indian Pediatr. 2016;53(Suppl 2):S157–8.
22. Khokhar S, Agrawal S, Gupta S, Gogia V, Agrawal T. Epidemiology of traumatic lenticular subluxation in India. Int Ophthalmol. 2014;34:197–204.
23. Shah MA, Shah SM, Shah SB, Patel CG, Patel UA. Morphology of traumatic cataract: does it play a role in final visual outcome? BMJ Open. 2011;1(1):e000060.

24. Singh RB, Thakur S, Ichhpujani P. BMJ Case Rep. 2018;11:e227465.
25. Roizen NJ, Mets MB, Blondis TA. Ophthalmic disorders in children with Down syndrome. Dev Med Child Neurol. 1994;36:594–600.
26. Bökenkamp A, Ludwig M. The oculocerebrorenal syndrome of Lowe: an update. Pediatr Nephrol. 2016;31:2201–12.
27. Mets MB. Eye manifestations of intrauterine infections. Ophthalmol Clin North Am. 2001;14:521–31.
28. Trumler AA. Evaluation of pediatric cataracts and systemic disorders. Curr Opin Ophthalmol. 2011;22:365–79.
29. Khokhar SK, Dhull C. Atlas of pediatric cataract. Springer Nature Singapore; 2019. p. 129.
30. He M, Wang D, Jiang Y. Overview of ultrasound biomicroscopy. J Curr Glaucoma Pract. 2012;6(1):25–53.
31. El Shakankiri NM, Bayoumi NH, Abdallah AH, El Sahn MM. Role of ultrasound and biomicroscopy in evaluation of anterior segment anatomy in congenital and developmental cataract cases. J Cataract Refract Surg. 2009;35:1893–905.
32. Deramo VA, Shah GK, Baumal CR, Fineman MS, Corrêa ZM, Benson WE, et al. The role of ultrasound biomicroscopy in ocular trauma. Trans Am Ophthalmol Soc. 1998;96:355–65.
33. Ohzeki T. The value of electrophysiological testing in assessment of visual function in children. Eur J Implant Refract Surg. 1990;2:249–52.
34. Capozzi P, Morini C, Piga S, Cuttini M, Vadalà P. Corneal curvature and axial length values in children with congenital/infantile cataract in the first 42 months of life. Invest Ophthalmol Vis Sci. 2008;49:4774–8.
35. Trivedi RH, Wilson ME. Keratometry in pediatric eyes with cataract. Arch Ophthalmol. 2008;126:38–42.
36. Trivedi RH, Wilson ME. Axial length measurements by contact and immersion techniques in pediatric eyes with cataract. Ophthalmology. 2011;118:498–502.
37. Wilson ME, Trivedi RH. Axial length measurement techniques in pediatric eyes with cataract. Saudi J Ophthalmol. 2012;26:13–7.
38. Tromans C, Haigh PM, Biswas S, et al. Accuracy of intraocular lens power calculation in paediatric cataract surgery. Br J Ophthalmol. 2001;85:939–41.
39. Vasavada V, Shah SK, Vasavada VA, Vasavada AR, Trivedi RH, Srivastava S, et al. Comparison of IOL power calculation formulae for pediatric eyes. Eye (Lond). 2016;30:1242–50.
40. Dahan E, Drusedau MU. Choice of lens and dioptric power in pediatricpseudophakia. J Cataract Refract Surg. 1997;23(Suppl 1):618–23.
41. Enyedi LB, Peterseim MW, Freedman SF, Buckley EG. Refractive changes after pediatric intraocular lens implantation. Am J Ophthalmol. 1998.
42. Khokhar SK, Tomar A, Pillay G, Agarwal E. Biometric changes in Indian pediatric cataract and postoperative refractive status. Indian J Ophthalmol. 2019;67:1068–72.
43. Agrawal S, Singh V, Vinod Kumar BM, Meena M, Srivastava RM, Katiyar V. Immediate sequential bilateral cataract surgery in children in a government medical university in India. J Clin Ophthalmol Res. 2020;8:14–7.
44. Dave H, Phoenix V, Becker ER, Lambert SR. Simultaneous vs sequential bilateral cataract surgery for infants with congenital cataracts: visual outcomes, adverse events, and economic costs. Arch Ophthalmol. 2010;128(8):1050–4.

Intraocular Lenses in Pediatric Patients

4

Vaishali Vasavada and Abhay R. Vasavada

4.1 Introduction

Intraocular lens (IOL) implantation is a standard practice in cataract surgery whether performed in an adult or child. It becomes even more important as the benefits with early correction of surgical aphakia in pediatric population cannot be overemphasized. As explained in previous chapters, IOL implantation in children can be a tricky preposition considering the dynamic nature of the evolving optical system. Multiple considerations including the type and power of IOL, associated ocular comorbidities, frequent need for additional procedures and occasional refractive surprises following pediatric cataract surgery makes the simple decision of IOL implantation somewhat complicated in children. Though spectacles and contact lenses too may be used to correct surgical aphakia, high dependency, associated economic burden, and cumbersome wearing of aphakia glasses make them less than ideal and emotionally taxing in small children.

This chapter aims to summarize views from recently published literature on various issues related to IOL implantation during cataract surgery in unilateral and bilateral pediatric cataracts, with a special focus on issues arising in developing countries. It will also help the reader in selection of appropriate IOL and achieve optimal outcomes in pediatric cataract surgery.

V. Vasavada (✉) · A. R. Vasavada
Raghudeep Eye Hospital Iladevi Cataract & IOL Research Centre, Ahmedabad, India
e-mail: vaishali@raghudeepeyeclinic.com; http://www.raghudeepeyehospital.com

S. Agrawal (ed.), *Pediatric Cataract*,
https://doi.org/10.1007/978-981-16-1736-2_4

4.2 Challenges in IOL Implantation in Children

Primary IOL implantation has the advantage of providing at least a partial optical correction at all times [1–4]. However, this benefit should be carefully weighed against the potential risks for intra as well as postoperative complications. IOL implantation in children older than 2 years of age is now an accepted practice worldwide, particularly in developing countries [5–7]. Surgeons are still cautious about implanting an IOL in infants keeping in mind the severity of the intraoperative and postoperative complications including exaggerated inflammatory response, high rate of visual axis obscuration (VAO), and secondary glaucoma. Furthermore, the benefit of primary IOL implantation may be lost in-case the desired postoperative refraction is not achieved. Numerous studies have pointed to unexpected refractive outcomes secondary to errors arising out of inaccurate biometry or unexpected axial length growth [8, 9]. Thus, primary IOL implantation in infants should be considered a choice only after due consideration to the potential risks (Table 4.1).

4.3 Selecting the Appropriate Patient

Selecting a suitable candidate for IOL implantation is necessary to ensure maximal success without increasing risks in children with cataract. It can be recommended on basis of literature and experience that normal sized eyes (>10 mm horizontal diameter) in infants 6 months and older should undergo IOL implantation as a primary procedure. Exceptions to this recommendation are associated ocular comorbidities (discussed later), limited surgical experience, nonavailability of appropriate implant and when in the bag implantation is not possible. In these situations secondary implantation may be better.

As will be discussed in detail later, the threshold age for IOL implantation in unilateral congenital cataracts (provided cataract is the only abnormality) is lower compared to bilateral cataracts considering the possibility of dense amblyopia in

Table 4.1 Benefits, risks, and challenges of IOL implantation in infants

Benefits
• Early visual rehabilitation with reduced spectacle dependence
• Reduced spectacle power translating to thinner, less heavy glasses
• Constant unaided visual input
Risks and challenges
• Higher risk of secondary procedures, particularly membranectomy
• Greater chances of inflammation/glaucoma with improper positioning of IOL
• Technically more demanding
• IOL power calculation and selection of target refraction difficult

these children from preoperative unilateral visual deprivation and severe postoperative anisometropia should these children be left aphakic.

Microcornea and microphthalmos are contraindications to *primary* IOL implantation, regardless of the age at surgery. Microcornea is usually defined as a horizontal corneal diameter of <9 mm, and microphthalmos is defined as an axial length (AL) which is less than 2 standard deviations of the reported normal AL for that age [8, 10]. Persistent fetal vasculature and juvenile/idiopathic arthritis, once considered as contraindications to IOL implantation are not absolute contraindications now due to better techniques and technology. However, in both these conditions, presence of microphthalmos, microcornea or severe, persistent, intractable uveitis may cause additional complications and these patients are better left aphakic in primary surgery (Table 4.2).

Secondary implantation of customized IOLs may be considered in microphthalmic eyes and in eyes with uveitis once the disease is controlled. However, these cases should be handled by experienced pediatric cataract surgeons.

Most cases of traumatic cataract barring a clean wound with minimal collateral injury, should undergo IOL implantation as a secondary procedure when appropriate assessment has been done and inflammation controlled.

The factors to be considered while planning for primary IOL implantation in children with unilateral or bilateral developmental cataracts are discussed in detail in the following sections.

4.3.1 IOL Implantation in Unilateral Developmental Cataract

In the 1970s, it was believed by ophthalmologists that unilateral cataracts should not be operated upon since they are associated with very poor visual prognosis [11]. Subsequently, it was established that cataract surgery in unilateral cataracts yields good outcomes [12–16]. Unilateral cataractous eyes may have comorbid conditions such as microphthalmos, persistent fetal vasculature, microcornea, and colobomas. Further, the amblyogenic potential of unilateral cataracts is greater than bilateral cataracts as explained in Chap. 1, and therefore timely surgery followed by intensive amblyopia treatment is required [5, 6, 17, 18]. Aphakic spectacles are practically not a viable option for these eyes due to significant aniseikonia associated with anisohypermetropia. Contact lenses are the only nonsurgical modality for optical

Table 4.2 Contraindications for primary IOL implantation in children

• Microphthalmos (Axial length ≤17 mm)
• Microcornea (Horizontal corneal diameter <9 mm)
• Inadequate anterior or posterior capsular support
• Uncontrolled glaucoma or uveitis
• Inexperienced surgeon
Relative contraindications
• Trauma
• Age below 6 months
• Juvenile idiopathic arthritis

correction of aphakia in these eyes. Advantages of contact lenses include the ability to change the contact lens power as needed to keep up with the rapidly growing eye's refractive needs, and avoiding spectacle wear during the first few years of life. However, the use of contact lenses in infants is challenging due to difficulty in insertion and removal of the lens, the complications involved in fitting the lens onto the steep cornea of infants and poor compliance. In developing countries, the repeated cost of replacing contact lenses due to frequent misplacement or damage as well as change in refraction is often a limiting factor. Limited parental education and hygiene levels also prohibit effective contact lens usage.

In infants there is still some controversy as to what should be the youngest age for implantation. Recent studies in the United States of America and by the British Isles Congenital Cataract Interest Group have found no added long-term visual benefit with primary IOL implantation in infants with added disadvantages of inflammatory sequelae, resurgeries, and anesthesia-related complications [19, 20]. However, it must be understood here that the control group (aphakic group) in these were compliant patients who used contact lenses. On the other hand, there have also been studies that report better visual acuity with primary IOL implantation as compared to primary aphakia [21–23].

Based on these and our experience, we recommend that primary IOL implantation in unilateral cataracts with normal-sized eyes should be performed in infants even below 6 months of age, except where regular and safe contact lens usage can be ensured.

Unilateral developmental cataracts carry an inherent risk of severe amblyopia and despite best efforts are prone to develop poor visual outcomes. Unilateral early-onset dense visual deprivation with abnormal binocular interaction due to anisometropia and loss of accommodation contributes to suboptimal results. Timely diagnosis, surgery as well as aggressive amblyopia therapy play a crucial role in improving visual acuity and regaining some binocular functions.

4.3.2 IOL Implantation in Bilateral Developmental Cataracts

Till a few years ago it was believed that spectacles for bilateral aphakia were compatible with good vision and secondary IOL implantation could be performed once the child grew up. But now it has been well demonstrated by other researchers and us that visual recovery is much faster when primary IOL implantation is performed, and the rates of serious postoperative complications are comparable after surgery in both groups (other group being children left aphakic) [24–27].

Thus, primary IOL implantation should be considered in infants with bilateral cataracts, wherever an in the bag IOL implantation can be performed.

4.4 IOL Power Determination in Pediatric Eyes

Implanting an IOL with appropriate refractive power is as important as selecting the right candidate for primary IOL implantation. Despite all efforts, predicting the axial growth of the eye and therefore, selecting an IOL of appropriate power for the eye is one of the biggest enigmas in pediatric cataract surgery. The following parameters play a crucial role in deciding the refractive power of an IOL.

4.4.1 Biometry

Precision in the measurement of axial length and corneal curvature is essential for accurate calculation of IOL power. Keratometry using a handheld keratometer performed under general anesthesia prior to surgery is the standard. This is followed by immersion ultrasound A scan for axial length measurement [28]. Older children may be cooperative on optical biometers. Published normative data may be used as an inferior alternative in normal-sized eyeballs where accuracy of measurements is doubtful. Implanting an IOL without biometry is not recommended. More details of biometry can be referred to in previous chapter on preoperative evaluation.

Several formulae, including the SRK-II, SRK-T, Hoffer Q, Holladay 1, Holladay 2, as well as Pediatric IOL Power calculator have been shown to be effective in IOL power calculation. However, achieving targeted refraction is often unpredictable [11, 29–34]. It appears that all modern IOL power calculation formulae (e.g. SRK/T, Holladay 2, Barrett Universal formula, Haigis) are more or less similar in their ability to achieve targeted refraction. Authors' recommendations are summarized in Table 4.3.

4.4.2 Target Postoperative Refraction

In addition to biometry, the power of IOL to be implanted is also determined by the targeted postsurgery refraction. This is typically considered in younger children in

Table 4.3 Preferred IOL formulae

Infants
• SRK/T or Holladay 2
Age 1–5 years
• SRK/T or Holladay 2
Age >5 years
• Barrett Universal
Secondary IOL implantation
• Barrett Universal

Table 4.4 Guidelines for undercorrection/postoperative refraction

IOL power-based on Axial Length [34]	
17 mm	25 D
18 mm	24 D
19 mm	23 D
20 mm	21 D
21 mm	19 D
Undercorrection based on SRK II formula [35]	
<6 months	20%
6 months to 1 year	15%
1 year	10%
2 years	5%
>5 years	None
Target postoperative refraction [36, 37]	
≤6 months	+10 to 6 D
6–12 months	+6 to 4 D
1–3 years	+4 D
3–6 years	+3 to 2 D
6–8 years	+1 to 0 D

whom the optical system is still evolving. Whether to aim for emmetropia or undercorrect the child in anticipation of a future myopic shift is debatable. The general consensus that should be followed by beginners, particularly for young children is to perform varying degrees of undercorrection (leaving behind residual hyperopic refractive error). In general, younger the child, more should be the undercorrection. Undercorrection may also be more in children with history of myopia in family. Undercorrection should be lesser in older children, unilateral surgery, and with anticipated poor compliance to optical correction or amblyopia therapy. Up to 30% under correction in calculated IOL power is practiced by many surgeons for children younger than 6 months with bilateral cataracts. Twenty percent undercorrection for children below 2 years and 10% under correction up to 8 years is also widely practiced [35]. It is important to strike a balance between the amblyogenic potential of postoperative residual hypermetropia and eventual myopia that would occur after completion of ocular growth.

General guidelines for target postoperative refraction/undercorrection based on published literature are summarized in Table 4.4 [34, 36, 37].

4.5 IOL Material, Type, and Size

Important consideration should also be given to the material of an IOL while considering primary or secondary IOL implantation to avoid postoperative complications. An appropriately sized IOL made out of a biocompatible material designed to provide good distant and near visual acuity would be ideal for implantation in children. Today, foldable hydrophobic acrylic IOLs with square edges have become the preferred IOL choice for most pediatric cataract surgeons [2, 3, 38–48] instead of the PMMA IOLs, which were once the IOLs of choice [44, 49, 50]. Being foldable, these IOLs offer all the benefits of smaller incision cataract surgery. Further, the hydrophobic acrylic material has excellent biocompatibility and is reported to cause lesser and more delayed posterior capsule opacification (PCO) [3, 47, 51]. Several reports regarding optimal outcome with standard hydrophilic IOLs in pediatric eyes also exist [47, 52, 53]. Heparin surface-modified rigid IOLs were in vogue, particularly when PMMA IOLs were preferred. Subsequently, some foldable hydrophilic lenses with heparin surface modification have become available. The rationale behind heparin passivated IOL was to reduce postoperative fierce inflammatory response in pediatric eyes. However, currently, due to better techniques, technology, and understanding to tackle postoperative inflammation, heparin surface-modified IOLs have limited availability and use. Using low-molecular weight heparin in the irrigating fluid to reduce postoperative inflammation in pediatric cataract surgery has equivocal reports [54, 55].

Another important issue in pediatric IOL implantation is the sizing of the IOL. Most IOLs available commercially have an overall diameter of 12.5–13 mm and an optic diameter of 5–6 mm, which are best suited for adult eyes. These IOLs may be too large for the pediatric capsular bag, especially when dealing with infants. Due to the limited use, smaller customized IOLs are expensive and only available on demand. While ordering customized IOL, the white to white corneal diameter and mesopic pupil are used to estimate the overall and optic size of the IOL, respectively. It should be remembered that microphthalmic eyes are only considered for secondary IOL implantation.

4.6 Additional Tips for IOL Implantation in Pediatric Cataract Surgery

While there are several differences between a successful pediatric cataract surgery and adult surgery the most significant amongst them is the management of posterior capsule. A posterior capsulotomy (manual/vitrectorhexis) is usually performed with or without anterior vitrectomy in children younger than 6 years. Therefore, special care needs to be taken in implanting IOLs in these eyes.

4.6.1 Preferred Site of IOL Implantation

The capsular bag is the preferred site of implantation the IOL (Fig. 4.1). A posterior capsulotomy may be performed prior to or following IOL implantation in the bag. Often, in infants and very young children, an IOL is implanted and subsequently either a manual posterior capsulorhexis (PCCC) is performed with or without anterior vitrectomy (through anterior approach), or a vitrectorhexis along with anterior vitrectomy is performed (through pars plana approach). This approach ensures that the IOL can be implanted in the bag safely without the risk of an inadvertently large PCCC that may endanger the bag placement. When implanting the IOL, care

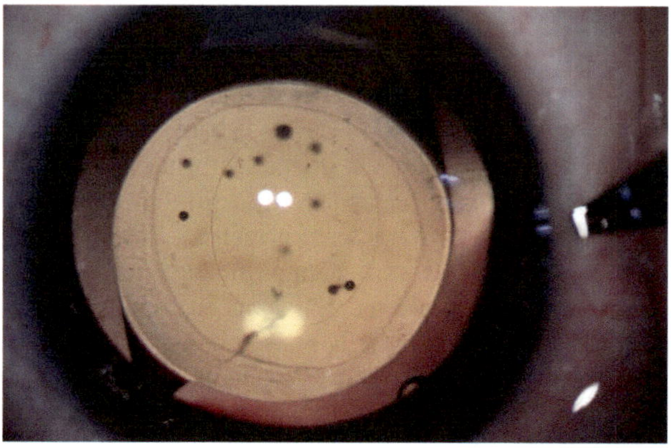

Fig. 4.1 Anterior and posterior manual capsulorhexes with in the bag placement of intraocular lens

should be taken to use an appropriate injector—cartridge system for the incision size. It may be better to enlarge the incision a little so as to make IOL implantation smooth and comfortable. Using a heavy molecular weight cohesive ophthalmic viscosurgical device (OVD) is helpful, since it keeps the capsular bag expanded. Choosing an IOL material and design that allows controlled, slow unfolding is preferred to enable easy positioning and to avoid inadvertent movement of the IOL through PCCC.

However, there are often situations where there may be preexisting or iatrogenic rupture in the posterior capsule. In this condition, it may become necessary to implant the IOL in the ciliary sulcus with or without capture of the IOL optic through the anterior and/or posterior capsulorhexes. Ciliary sulcus implantation of IOL should be performed only in the event of a posterior capsule rupture or inadvertently large PCCC that precludes in the bag implantation.

4.6.2 Optic Capture of IOL

In the technique of optic capture, first described for pediatric eyes by Howard Gimbel [56], an IOL is placed in the capsular bag following anterior and posterior capsulorhexes, and thereafter, the IOL optic is slid behind the PCCC margin, so as to "lock it" in position (Fig. 4.2). This ensures both, IOL stability as well as retardation of VAO since the fusion of anterior and posterior capsulorhexes margins prevents central migration of proliferating lens epithelial cells. Optic capture of IOL has been discussed in detail in the next chapter.

Visual axis obscuration (VAO) is one of the biggest hurdles for visual rehabilitation following successful pediatric cataract surgery (Fig. 4.3), particularly when surgery is performed at a young age [57–63]. To overcome this, PCCC with anterior vitrectomy has become an integral part of the surgical strategy for young children. However, with optic capture VAO can be delayed or reduced without anterior vitrectomy as has been shown by us in a recent randomized study [64].

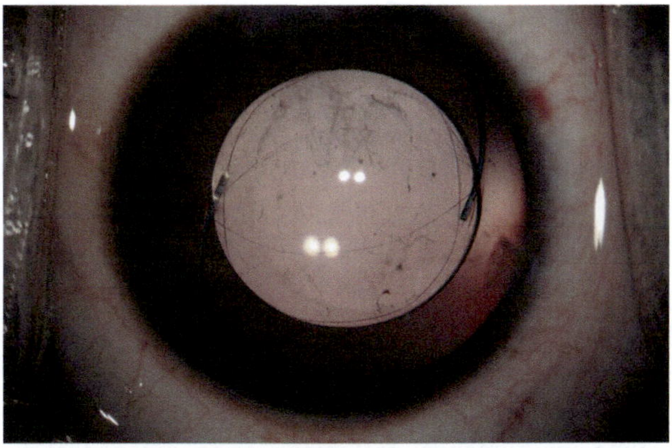

Fig. 4.2 Three piece foldable intraocular lens placed in the capsular bag and the optic captured through the posterior capsulorhexis

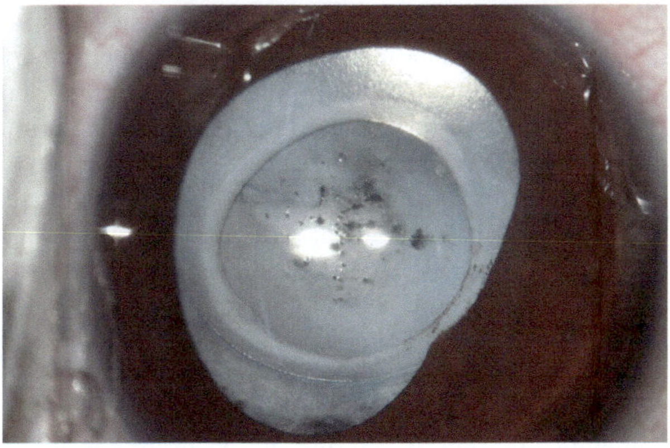

Fig. 4.3 Dense visual axis obscuration caused by proliferation of residual lens epithelial cells following pediatric cataract surgery

4.6.3 Toric and Multifocal IOLs

Preexisting corneal astigmatism is a problem in both adult and pediatric cataract surgery. Further, astigmatism has the potential to cause meridional amblyopia in the pediatric population. Since toric IOLs have been largely successful in adult eyes, surgeons have started adopting the use of these IOLs to deal with preexisting corneal astigmatism even in pediatric eyes. Although, there are not many reports in literature, the technology appears promising by aiming to correct one of the amblyogenic factors in the growing population [65, 66]. However, it is important that only children older than 5 years with reliable biometry and corneal topography be selected for toric IOL implantation as the corneal curvature only stabilizes by 5–6 years of age.

Multifocal IOLs have the advantage of reducing spectacle dependence at all distances. However, with all currently available designs of multifocal IOLs, most of which have diffractive optics, there is a variable reduction of light transmission to the retina, which inherently reduces contrast sensitivity and can give rise to dysphotopic phenomena. In the developing visual system, reduction of contrast and the quality of vision would be more detrimental and amblyogenic overshadowing the theoretical advantage of spectacle independence. Further, since these are growing eyes, the refraction and axial growth are dynamic and changing. The issues related to decentration and IOL power calculation also get exaggerated with these lenses. Although there are some reports of their use in pediatric eyes [67, 68], presently it is not recommended to perform multifocal IOL implantation in pediatric cataract surgery [69].

4.6.4 Secondary IOL Implantation

Children are sometimes left aphakic during their primary surgery, either due to young age, surgeons' preference, or conditions that preclude primary IOL implantation (Table 4.2). Secondary IOL implantation is a feasible option once the child grows up, and more importantly, the eye achieves an AL and corneal diameter suitable for IOL implantation. Most surgeons prefer to perform secondary IOL implantation when the child is about 3 years old or when the corneal diameter and AL grow to the normal size for the child's age. During the primary surgery when the young child is left aphakic, meticulous care should be taken to appropriately size the anterior and posterior capsulorhexes along with complete cortical removal, to ensure adequate capsular support for future IOL implantation.

In the secondary surgery, the IOL can be placed in the capsular bag or in the ciliary sulcus [70, 71], but in the bag implantation is preferable as it causes lower inflammation postoperatively. In the bag, IOL placement requires the surgeon to open up the fused capsules and create space in the capsular bag. Although ideal, this surgical strategy is challenging and may not be always possible due to near-complete adhesion of anterior and posterior capsules. In this situation, the IOL is implanted in the ciliary sulcus, and the optic is captured through the capsulorhexis opening if the rhexis size allows. It should be kept in mind that only three-piece foldable IOLs should be implanted in the ciliary sulcus. Sulcus implantation of single-piece foldable IOLs causes inflammation and/or glaucoma [72]. After secondary IOL implantation, close followup should be maintained for postoperative inflammation, glaucoma, and retinal complications.

4.7 Summary

- Primary in the bag IOL implantation should be performed in children above 6 months of age with no other comorbid condition in the eye.
- Implantation should be performed after meticulous biometry.
- SRK/T or Holladay 1 formulae are used in children below 5 years of age.
- Under correction from the calculated emmetropic power should be done to compensate for the growth of the eye.
- Lesser under correction is done in older children, unilateral surgery, and in those with anticipated poor compliance to optical correction or amblyopia therapy.

- Foldable hydrophobic acrylic IOLs are the first choice.
- Toric and multifocal IOLs are not recommended in children.
- Secondary IOL implantation is done at about 3 years of age in children left aphakic at the time of primary surgery.

Multiple Choice Questions

1. Contraindications for primary IOL implantation in pediatric eyes include:
   (a) Microphthalmos
   (b) Microcornea
   (c) Uncontrolled juvenile arthritis
   (d) All of the above

   Answer: *d. All of the above*. Primary IOL implantation is contraindicated in all these conditions.

2. Which method is preferred in infant's eyes for axial length measurement?
   (a) Contact A scan ultrasound
   (b) B scan ultrasound
   (c) Immersion A scan ultrasound
   (d) Optical biometer

   Answer: c. *Immersion A scan ultrasound*. Contact A scan and B scan are inaccurate. They cause indentation and result in lesser than actual measurements. Immersion A scan should be performed preferably under anesthesia, prior to surgery. Infants are not expected to cooperate on optical biometer.

3. Which IOL material is preferred for IOL implantation in pediatric eyes?
   (a) Silicone
   (b) Hydrophobic acrylic
   (c) Polymethyl Methacrylate (PMMA)
   (d) Both A and C

   Answer: *b. Hydrophobic acrylic*. Hydrophobic acrylic foldable IOLs are preferred in pediatric eyes. Silicone lenses have a higher incidence of posterior capsule opacification. PMMA lenses are rigid and non-foldable.

4. What complications should be looked for postoperatively following IOL implantation in pediatric eyes?
   (a) Glaucoma
   (b) Visual axis obscuration (VAO)
   (c) Inflammation
   (d) All of the above

   Answer: *d. All of the above*. All these complications may occur after IOL implantation in children more frequently than in adults.

5. Which is the preferred site for IOL implantation in pediatric eyes?
   (a) Capsular bag
   (b) Ciliary sulcus
   (c) Anterior chamber
   (d) Scleral fixation

   Answer: *a. Capsular bag*. Capsular bag implantation places the IOL in the most physiological position. It also causes the least complications like decentration and inflammation.

References

1. Lambert SR, Lynn M, Drews-Botsch C, et al. A comparison of grating visual acuity, strabismus and reoperation outcomes among children with aphakia and pseudophakia after unilateral cataract surgery within the first 6 months of life. J AAPOS. 2001;5:70–5.
2. Plager D, Yang S, Neely D, et al. Complications in the first year following cataract surgery with and without IOL in infants and older children. J AAPOS. 2002;6:9–14.
3. Trivedi RH, Wilson ME Jr, Bartholomew LR, et al. Opacification of the visual axis after cataract surgery and single acrylic intraocular lens implantation in the first year of life. J AAPOS. 2004;8:156–64.
4. Tuncer S, Gucukoglu A, Gozum N. Cataract extraction and primary hydrophobic acrylic intraocular lens implantation in infants. J AAPOS. 2005;9:250–6.
5. Ruth AL, Lambert SR. Amblyopia in the phakic eye after unilateral congenital cataract extraction. J AAPOS. 2006;10:587–8.
6. Lewis TL, Maurer D, Brent HP. Development of grating acuity in children treated for unilateral or bilateral congenital cataract. Invest Ophthal Vis Sci. 1995;36:2080–95.
7. Allen RJ, Speedwell L, Russell-Eggit I. Long-term visual outcome after extraction of unilateral congenital cataracts. Eye. 2010;24:1263–7.
8. Lambert SR, Lynn MJ, Hartmann EE, et al. Comparison of contact lens and intraocular lens correction of monocular aphakia during infancy: a randomized clinical trial of HOTV optotype acuity at age 4.5 years and clinical findings at age 5 years. JAMA Ophthalmol. 2014;132:676–82.
9. Lambert SR, Lynn MJ, DuBois LG, Cotsonis GA, Hartmann EE, Wilson ME, Infant Aphakia Treatment Study Groups. Axial elongation following cataract surgery during the first year of life in the infant Aphakia Treatment Study. Invest Ophthalmol Vis Sci. 2012;53(12):7539–45.
10. Hoffman RS, Vasavada AR, Allen QB, et al. for the ASCRS Cataract Clinical Committee, Challenging/Complicated Cataract Surgery Subcommittee. Cataract surgery in the small eye. J Cataract Refract Surg. 2015;41:2565–75.
11. Sukhija J, Kaur S, Ram J. Outcome of a new acrylic intraocular lens implantation in pediatric cataract. J Pediatr Ophthalmol Strabismus. 2015;52:371–6.
12. Hubel DH, Weisel TN. Receptive fields of cells in striate cortex of very young, visually unexperienced kittens. J Neurophysiol. 1963;26:994–1002.
13. Hubel DH, Weisel TN. Effects of monocular deprivation in kittens. Naunyn Schmeidebergs Arch Exp Pathol Pharmakol. 1964;248:492–7.
14. Weisel TN, Hubel DH. Effects of visual deprivation on morphology and physiology of cells in the cat's lateral geniculate body. J Neurophysiol. 1963;26:978–93.
15. Weisel TN, Hubel DH. Single-cell responses in striate cortex of kittens deprived of vision in one eye. J Neurophysiol. 1963;26:1003–17.
16. Frey T, Friendly D, Wyatt D. Re-evaluation of monocular cataracts in children. Am J Ophthalmol. 1973;76:381–8.

17. Reese AB. Persistent hyperplastic primary vitreous. The Edward Jackson Memorial Lecture. Am J Ophthalmol. 1955;40:317–31.
18. Lundvall A, Kugelberg U. Outcome after treatment of congenital unilateral cataract. Acta Ophthalmol Scand. 2002;80:588092.
19. Day AC, MacLaren RE, Bruce C, et al. Outcomes of phacoemulsification and intraocular lens implantation in microphthalmos and nanophthalmos. J Cataract Refract Surg. 2013;39:87–96.
20. Infant Aphakia Treatment Study Group. Comparison of contact lens and intraocular lens correction of monocular aphakia during infancy: a randomized clinical trial of HOTV optotype acuity at age 4.5 years and clinical findings at 5 years. JAMA Ophthalmol. 2014;132:676–82.
21. Solebo AL, Russell-Eggitt I, Cumberland PM, Rahi JS. British Isles Congenital Cataract interest group. Risks and outcomes associated with primary intraocular lens implantation in children under 2 years of age: the IoL under 2 cohort study. Br J Ophthalmol. 2015;99:1471–6.
22. Lambert SR, Lynn M, Drews-Botsch C, et al. Optotype acuity and re-operation rate after unilateral cataract surgery within the first 6 months of life with or without IOL implantation. Br J Ophthalmol. 2004;88:1387–90.
23. Kumar P, Lambert SR. Evaluating the evidence for and against the use of IOLs in infants and young children. Expert Rev Med Devices. 2016;13:381–9.
24. Magli A, Forte R, Carrelli R, et al. Longterm outcomes of primary intraocular lens implantation for unilateral congenital cataracts. Seminophthalmol. 2015;21:1–6.
25. Vasavada AR, Vasavada V, Shah SK, et al. Five-year postoperative outcomes of bilateral Aphakia and Pseudophakia in children up to 2 years of age: a randomized clinical trial. Am J Ophthalmol. 2018;193:33–44.
26. Gupta A, Kekunnaya R, Ramappa M, Vaddavalli PK. Br J Ophthalmol. 2011;95:477–80.
27. Struck MC. Long-term results of pediatric cataract surgery and primary intraocular lens implantation from 7 to 22 months of life. JAMA Ophthalmol. 2015;133:1180–3.
28. Wilson ME Jr, Trivedi RH. Eye growth after pediatric cataract surgery. Am J Ophthalmol. 2004;138:1039–40.
29. Fan DS, Rao SK, Yu CB, et al. Changes in refraction and ocular dimensions after cataract surgery and primary intraocular lens implantation in infants. J Cataract Refract Surg. 2006;32:1104–8.
30. Nihalani BR, VanderVeen DK. Comparison of intraocular lens power calculation formulae in pediatric eyes. Ophthalmology. 2010;117(8):1493–9.
31. Vanderveen DK, Nizam A, Lynn MJ, et al. Predictability of intraocular lens power calculation and early refractive status: the Infant Aphakia Treatment Study. Arch Ophthalmol. 2012;130:293–9.
32. Vanderveen DK, Trivedi RH, Nizam A, et al. Predictability of intraocular lens power calculation formulae in infantile eyes with unilateral congenital cataract: results from the Infant Aphakia Treatment Study. Am J Ophthalmol. 2013;156:1252–60.
33. Trivedi RH, Wilson ME, Reardon W. Accuracy of the Holladay 2 intraocular lens for pediatric eyes in the absence of preoperative refraction. J Cataract Refract Surg. 2011;37:1239–43.
34. Vasavada V, Shah SK, Vasavada VA, et al. Comparison of IOL power calculation formulae for pediatric eyes. Eye. 2016;30:1242–50.
35. Dahan E, Drusedau MU. Choice of lens and dioptric power in pediatric pseudophakia. J Cataract Refract Surg. 1997;23(Suppl 1):618–23.
36. Khokhar SK, Tomar A, Pillay G, Agarwal E. Response to comments on Biometric changes in Indian pediatric cataract and postoperative refractive status. Indian J Ophthalmol. 2019;67:1907.
37. Enyedi LB, Peterseim MW, Freeman SF, Buckley EG. Refractive changes after pediatric intraocular lens implantation. Am J Ophthalmol. 1998;126:772–81.
38. Serafino M, Trivedi RH, Levin AV, et al. Use of the Delphi process in paediatric cataract management. Br J Ophthalmol. 2016;100(5):611–5.
39. Vasavada AR, Nath VC, Trivedi RH. Anterior vitreous face behavior with Acrysof in pediatric cataract surgery. J AAPOS. 2003;7:384–8.

40. Vasavada AR, Trivedi RH, Nath VC. Visual axis opacification after Acrysof intraocular lens implantation in children. J Cataract Refract Surg. 2004;30:1073–81.
41. Dahan E. Implantation in children. Curr Opinion Ophthalmol. 2000;11:51–5.
42. Stagner DR Jr, Weakly DR Jr, Hunter LS. Long term rates of PCO following small incision foldable acrylic intraocular lens implantation in children. J Pediatr Ophthalmol Strabismus. 2003;39:73–6.
43. Kugelberg M, Zetterstorm C. Pediatric cataract surgery with or without vitrectomy. J Cataract Refract Surg. 2002;28:1770–3.
44. Ram J, Brar S, Kaushik S. Role of posterior capsulotomy with vitrectomy and intraocular lens design and material in reducing posterior capsule opacification after pediatric cataract surgery. J Cataract Refract Surg. 2003;29:1579–84.
45. Rowe NA, Biswas S, Lloyd IC. Primary IOL implantation in children. A risk analysis of foldable acrylic versus PMMA lenses. J Cataract Refract Surg. 2004;88:481–5.
46. Raina UK, Mehta DK, Monga S, et al. Functional outcomes of acrylic intraocular lenses in pediatric cataract surgery. J Cataract Refract Surg. 2004;30:1082–91.
47. Trivedi RH, Wilson ME Jr. Single piece acrylic intraocular lens implantation in children. J Cataract Refract Surg. 2003;29:1738–43.
48. Kugelberg M, Kugelberg U, Bobrova N, et al. After cataract in children having cataract surgery with or without anterior vitrectomy implanted with a single piece Acrysof intraocular lens. J Cataract Refract Surg. 2005;31:757–62.
49. Ram J, Jain VK, Agarwal A, Kumar J. Hydrophobic acrylic versus polymethyl methacrylate intraocular lens implantation following cataract surgery in the first year of life. Graefes Arch Clin Exp Ophthalmol. 2014;252:1443–9.
50. Wilson ME, Trivedi RH. Choice of intraocular lens for pediatric cataract surgery: survey of AAPOS members. J Cataract Refract Surg. 2007;33:1666–7.
51. Linebarger EJ, Hardten DR, Shah GK, Lindstrom RL. Phacoemulsification and modern cataract surgery. Surv Ophthalmol. 1999;44:123–47.
52. Sen P, Kshetrapal M, Shah C, Mohan A, Jain E, Sen A. Posterior capsule opacification rate after phacoemulsification in pediatric cataract: hydrophilic versus hydrophobic intraocular lenses. J Cataract Refract Surg. 2019;45(10):1380–5.
53. Adhikari S, Shrestha UD. Pediatric cataract surgery with hydrophilic acrylic intraocular lens implantation in Nepalese children. Clin Ophthalmol. 2017;12:7–11.
54. Bayramlar H, Totan Y, Borazan M. Heparin in the intraocular irrigating solution in pediatric cataract surgery. J Cataract Refract Surg. 2004;30(10):2163–9. https://doi.org/10.1016/j.jcrs.2004.07.003.
55. Vasavada VA, Praveen MR, Shah SK, et al. Anti-inflammatory effects of low-molecular weight heparin in pediatric cataract surgery: a randomized, clinical trial. Am J Ophthalmol. 2012;154:252–8.
56. Gimbel HV. Posterior continuous curvilinear capsulorhexis and optic capture of the intraocular lens to prevent secondary opacification in pediatric cataract surgery. J Cataract Refract Surg. 1997;23:652–6.
57. Lambert SR, Buckley EG, Drews-Botsch CD, et al. Infant Aphakia Treatment Study Group. The infant aphakia treatment study: design and clinical measures at enrolment. Arch Ophthalmol. 2010;128:21–7.
58. Plager DA, Yang S, Neely D, Sprunger D, Sondhi N. Complications in the first year following cataract surgery with and without IOL in infants and older children. J AAPOS. 2002;6:9–14.
59. Lambert SR, Lynn M, Drews-Botsch C, Loupe D, Plager DA, Medow NB, Wilson ME, Buckley EG, Drack AV, Fawcett SL. A comparison of grating visual acuity, strabismus, and reoperation outcomes among children with aphakia and pseudophakia after unilateral cataract surgery during the first six months of life. J AAPOS. 2001;5:70–5.
60. BenEzra D, Cohen E. Posterior capsulectomy in pediatric cataract surgery; the necessity of a choice. Ophthalmology. 1997;104:2168–74.
61. Apple DJ, Solomon KD, Tetz MR, et al. Posterior capsule opacification. Surv Ophthalmol. 1992;37:73–116.

62. Koch DD, Kohnen T. A retrospective comparison of techniques to prevent secondary cataract formation following posterior chamber intraocular lens implantation in infants and children. Trans Am Ophthalmol Soc. 1997;95:351–60.
63. McDonnell PJ, Zarbin MA, Green WR. Posterior capsule opacification cification in pseudophakic eyes. Ophthalmology. 1983;90:1548–53.
64. Vasavada AR, Vasavada V, Shah SK, et al. Postoperative outcomes of intraocular lens implantation in the bag versus posterior optic capture in pediatric cataract surgery. J Cataract Refract Surg. 2017;43:1177–83.
65. Ram J, Singh R, Gupta R, et al. Toric intraocular lens implantation in children with developmental cataract and preexisting corneal astigmatism. Acta Ophthalmologica. 2017;95:e95–e100.
66. Gimbel HV, Camoriano GD, Aman-Ullah M. Bilateral implantation of scleral-fixated cionniendocapsular rings and toric intraocular lenses in a pediatric patient with Marfan's syndrome. Case Rep Ophthalmol. 2012;3:16–23.
67. Jacobi PC, Dietlein TS, Konen W. Multifocal intraocular lens implantation in pediatric cataract surgery. Ophthalmology. 2001;108(8):1375–80.
68. Abouzeid H, Moetteli L, Munier FL. New-generation multifocal intraocular lens for pediatric cataract. Ophthalmologica. 2013;230:100–7.
69. Braga-Mele R, Chang D, Dewey S, et al. (ASCRS Cataract Clinical Committee). Multifocal intraocular lenses: relative indications and contraindications for implantation. J Cataract Refract Surg. 2014;40:313–22.
70. Nihalani B, Vanderween DK. Secondary intraocular lens implantation after pediatric aphakia. J AAPOS. 2011;15:435–40.
71. Wilson ME, Hafez GA, Trivedi RH. Secondary in – the – bag – intraocular lens implantation in children who have been aphakic since early infancy. JAAPOS. 2011;15:162–6.
72. Vasavada AR, Raj SM, Karve S, et al. Retrospective ultrasound biomicroscopic analysis of single-piece sulcus-fixated acrylic intraocular lenses. J Cataract Refract Surg. 2010;36:771–7.

Pediatric Cataract Surgery

5

Siddharth Agrawal, Rajat M. Srivastava, and Nitika Pandey

5.1 Introduction

Pediatric cataract surgery is challenging even for experienced cataract surgeons not only because of the smaller size of the eye but also because of the physiological dissimilarities from the adult eye. To be able to perform the surgery with competency it is recommended that where possible, pediatric cataract surgery should be done by surgeons who perform it on a weekly or biweekly basis [1]. This, however, is not possible in small practices and may also result in unnecessary delay in management. All steps require special care including incisions, capsulorhexis, intraocular lens injection, posterior capsule and anterior vitreous management. This chapter describes the steps of cataract surgery in pediatric eyes, highlights their differences from those in adults and helps the occasional pediatric cataract surgeon avoid complications.

5.2 Challenges with Pediatric Cataract Surgery

A good surgery is one of the most important steps in management of pediatric cataract. Pediatric eye poses unique challenges in management of cataract. A surgeon must be well aware of them before embarking on to pediatric cataract surgery. Some of the challenges routinely encountered while managing pediatric cataracts are mentioned here.

S. Agrawal (✉) · R. M. Srivastava · N. Pandey
Department of Ophthalmology, King George's Medical University, Lucknow, India

S. Agrawal (ed.), *Pediatric Cataract*,
https://doi.org/10.1007/978-981-16-1736-2_5

5.2.1 Need for General Anaesthesia

While adult cataract surgery is routinely performed under topical anaesthesia, any ocular procedure in children requires general anaesthesia (GA). For an anaesthetist this requires evaluation of systemic fitness and the operating team needs to be prepared for even the less frequently required procedures in all cases. The surgeon should also be meticulous in each step as a detailed post-operative examination is difficult in uncooperative children. The details related to anaesthesia have been discussed later in the chapter.

5.2.2 Decreased Scleral Rigidity

Decreased scleral rigidity and tendency of children to rub the eyes may cause the incisions to gape. Even corneal incision is less likely to self-seal in children compared to adults [2]. For this reason, suturing of all the wounds, including the paracentesis with 10-0 nylon or 10-0 vicryl suture is recommended.

5.2.3 Lesser Space in Anterior Chamber and Capsular Bag

Smaller eyes imply lesser space for manipulation, more chance of inadvertent injury to corneal endothelium and difficulty in appropriate placement of intraocular lens (IOL). Preoperative estimates of the white to white diameter and axial length are essential to decide about the implantation of IOL. It is estimated that the size of the capsular bag changes from 7.0 mm at birth to 9.0 mm at 2 years of age [3].

As discussed in the previous chapter, IOL implantation is comfortable in normal-sized eyes (>10.0 mm corneal diameter) in infants over 6 months of age, the surgeon should be adequately cautious in small eyes with corneal diameter <9.5 mm. It is better to leave these infants aphakic initially. Customized small IOLs may be considered in microphthalmic eyes of children over 2 years of age since growth of the eye is almost complete by then [4]. Placing an adult-sized IOL in a small eye will only have disastrous consequences.

Small, non-dilating pupils are common in infants and more so in cataracts associated with rubella. Use of ophthalmic visco-surgical devices (OVD), iris hooks or certain special techniques may be required to proceed safely.

5.2.4 Capsular Elasticity

Pediatric capsules (both anterior and posterior) are elastic, resist tearing and get stretched making the continuous curvilinear capsulorhexis (CCC) difficult. It has been found that the anterior capsule extensibility is maximal in infancy and decreases by about 0.5% per year throughout life [5]. Several options of achieving successful CCC have been discussed in the chapter.

5.2.5 Anterior Chamber Instability

Non-self-sealing nature of the incisions, lesser space in the anterior chamber and increased vitreous thrust make the anterior chamber prone to collapse making the surgery difficult. The use of higher viscosity cohesive OVDs is essential to maintain chamber stability.

5.2.6 Lens Aspiration Only

The lens matter is usually soft and flows out after hydration. The cortex can be easily aspirated manually (with Simcoe bimanual cannula) or with phaco irrigation aspiration handpiece. Exceptions to this are some rubella cataracts (which often have a calcified capsule and nucleus) and fibrotic membranes of persistent fetal vasculature (PFV).

5.2.7 Increased Inflammation

The eyes of children react with greater inflammation post-operatively compared to adults even after a satisfactory surgery [6]. This is due to immaturity of the blood–aqueous barrier in pediatric eyes [7]. The intraocular inflammation is greater and prolonged when the iris requires manipulation (e.g. small pupil and trauma), cortical clean-up is inadequate or the IOL is implanted in the sulcus. Anterior chamber cells, flare, fibrinous reaction and posterior synechiae occur in the early post-operative period. Synechiae formation, visual axis opacification, pupillary capture and pigmentation over the IOL are frequent long-term consequences of this inflammation [8, 9]. Several measures are undertaken to minimize the inflammation and its consequences, which have been discussed later.

The compact vitreous gel makes the pediatric eyes protective to cystoid macular oedema [10].

5.2.8 The Growing Globe

The changing refractive properties of the cornea and crystalline lens along with the increasing axial length of the eye make decision about the IOL power a challenge. This has been discussed at several places in the earlier chapters.

5.2.9 Visual Axis Opacification

Increased proliferation of lens epithelial cells (LEC) and increased inflammation make the pediatric eyes more prone to visual axis opacification (VAO). Anterior vitreous face is more closely linked to the posterior capsule which acts as a scaffold

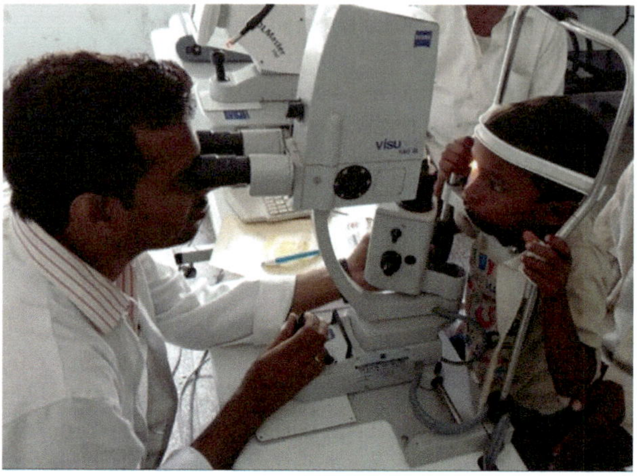

Fig. 5.1 Children as young as 4 years may cooperate for YAG laser capsulotomy

for proliferating LECs and metaplastic pigment cells. Thorough cortical clean up, proper IOL choice and placement, primary management of posterior capsule and anterior vitreous, appropriate cycloplegics and anti-inflammatory medications prevent or delay the formation of VAO. Heparin surface-modified IOLs, use of heparin (5 IU/ml) in irrigating fluid and use of tissue plasminogen activator reduce the formation of fibrin and secondary membranes [11, 12].

VAO is the commonest late post-operative complication and when significant requires surgical management in small children. Children over 4 years of age may be cooperative for laser capsulotomy which should be attempted before the opacification becomes thick (Fig. 5.1).

Planning cataract surgery in children thus requires special attention to unique challenges it presents. In the following sections, we discuss in detail, the relevant concerns encountered while planning and performing pediatric cataract surgery.

5.3 Preoperative Planning

Preoperative evaluation, decision-making and counselling have been dealt in the earlier chapters. We mention the important points here.

5.3.1 When to Operate?

It should be clearly understood that every lenticular opacity does not warrant surgery. Small central opacities (<3 mm) and larger peripheral opacities (frequently after trauma) can be managed by refraction and prescription of appropriate correction [13]. A visual acuity of 6/9 (LogMAR 0.17) with crystalline lens and preserved accommodation is far better than that of 6/6 (LogMAR 0.0) with an artificial lens. Such children should be kept under follow ups and observed for progression of cataract. Appropriate parent counselling is essential.

Central cataracts larger than 3 mm, those closer to the nodal point (posterior cataracts), obscuring retinal examination or retinoscopy, causing nystagmus or strabismus can be considered to be visually significant. They should be managed as early as possible in infancy, possibly as soon as the child is fit for general anaesthesia. All unilateral developmental cataracts should be managed before 4–6 weeks and bilateral before 6–8 weeks of age preferably [14, 15]. The urgency of management is greater in unilateral cataracts due to their greater amblyogenic potential as discussed in Chap. 1. It is for the same reason that in symmetrical bilateral cases, the second eye should be operated within a week after the first and may even be operated in the same sitting in children at higher risk for general anaesthesia [16, 17]. In presence of significant asymmetry, the denser cataract is usually operated first. Prognosis for visual recovery becomes guarded once nystagmus or searching movements develop, usually at about 13 weeks in untreated cataract [18, 19].

Children presenting with trauma may undergo primary or secondary management of cataract depending on the condition of other ocular tissues and presence of inflammation as discussed in Chap. 7.

5.3.2 Informed Consent

Informed consent from the parents/legal guardians is the most important step of preoperative counselling. The procedure, its benefits and possible complications should be explained and the attendants should be given time to clarify their doubts. Adolescent patients should be encouraged to participate. They should also sign an informed assent besides the consent given by their parents. The treating team should realize that few minutes spent preoperatively in counselling are more effective than several hours spent after the surgery. The discussion should be tailored to individual patients, the attitude should be sympathetic and the message unambiguous. Adequate time should be given and the decision should be respected.

Informed consent form used by us for pediatric cataract surgery is available as Annexure 1 at the end of this chapter. This has been adapted from the recommendations of the All India Ophthalmological Society [20]. The reader must remember that separate consents would be required for (1) general anaesthesia and (2) in patients of trauma.

5.3.3 Intraocular Lens

Several issues related to IOL have to be addressed prior to surgery like whether to implant, which implant to use and the power of the implant. These have been addressed in Chaps. 3 and 4.

5.3.4 Surgical Options

Decisions about the instrumentation (lens aspiration or lensectomy), approach (anterior or pars plana), posterior capsule management and anterior vitrectomy have to be made prior to surgery. These have been covered in relevant sections below.

5.4 Preoperative Preparation

Mydriasis and cycloplegia are achieved by use of 2% homatropine eye drops 1 day prior to surgery or 1% atropine eye ointment twice daily for 3 days preoperatively. A tiny amount of ointment should be used each time to minimize the systemic side effects. Flurbiprofen (0.03%) eye drops twice at 10-min interval preoperatively helps in sustaining the mydriasis [21].

Children should also receive topical 0.3% tobramycin or 0.5% moxifloxacin four times a day (t/d) for 3 days preoperatively and one drop of 5% betadine solution immediately preoperatively as prophylaxis [22].

To shrink the vitreous volume 1–2 g/kg of intravenous mannitol may be given over 30–60 min, especially in children who are to undergo posterior capsulotomy.

It should be ensured that the instructions given by the anaesthesia team including keeping the child nil orally are followed sincerely. The parents should be advised to keep a watch and inform the operating team if the child consumes food or water in the hours prior to surgery.

Checklist for receiving the patient in operating room is given as Annexure 2.

5.5 General Anaesthesia

Most pediatric cataract surgeries are performed under GA. Due to inherent risks involved in GA, it is essential to be well prepared to ensure safety and to minimize the exposure to GA.

5.5.1 Preoperative Assessment

While most children with developmental cataract are otherwise medically fit, the anaesthetist should be aware of the systemic conditions which may be associated. Intubation may be difficult in cataracts associated with mucopolysaccharidoses and thromboembolism may be associated with homocystinuria. Prophylactic treatment with aspirin in consultation with a pediatrician may be considered preoperatively in patients of homocystinuria. Children with cataract associated with maternal rubella may have congenital heart defects and may develop apnoea during induction or extubation.

The anaesthesia team should also have a sympathetic attitude towards these children who are unable to see and are unaware of their surroundings. Simple measures like using an anaesthetic cream on the dorsum of the hand before intravenous (iv) cannulation prevents pain, associated crying and possible oxygen desaturation in children with compromised circulation [23]. Many systemic (chromosomal and metabolic) abnormalities are associated with mental retardation and even older children may not understand the instructions being given.

Pediatric cataract surgeries often take longer than expected due to additional procedures like vitrectomy that may not have been initially planned, and the anaesthesia team should be prepared for it. It is also for this reason that local anaesthesia should not be considered in older, otherwise cooperative children who may have even a remote requirement of posterior capsule management (e.g. in presence of trauma).

5.5.2 Special Considerations in Pediatric Patients

The components of anaesthesia are unconsciousness (with amnesia), analgesia and muscle relaxation (diminished responses). Smooth induction and reversal are also desirable in all surgeries, more so in intraocular surgeries in children. The temperature of the room should be regulated and the child should be kept warm. Infants are especially prone to develop hypothermia. While details of pediatric anaesthesia are outside the scope of this book, we highlight here some practical tips which may be of interest and concern to the surgeon as well.

Having a secure airway is essential as the face is covered with drape during the surgery and access to it by the anaesthesia team is restricted. While earlier it was recommended to perform tracheal intubation in children and to use a reinforced flexible tracheal tube in infants below 6 months of age, now it has been shown that pressure-controlled ventilation using laryngeal mask is effective and safe [24]. Fears of gastric insufflation and reflux are unfounded. The laryngeal mask also offers the advantage of smoother extubation with lesser coughing and thereby reduces the chances of acute increase of intraocular pressure (IOP) during its removal, compared to conventional tracheal extubation [25].

The tubes should be clamped on the opposite side of the eye being operated or vertically down and the anaesthesia team should move towards the foot end of the patient after securing the airway, reconfirming the iv access and attaching the electrodes, leaving the upper half of the patient clear for the surgical team.

The anaesthetist should be aware of the drugs used preoperatively for mydriasis. Commonly used are parasympatholytic agents like atropine or cyclopentolate and sympathomimetic ones like phenylephrine. They may be supplemented intraoperatively if adequate mydriasis has not been achieved. Though safe, they may cause serious side effects like hypertension and pulmonary oedema if systemically absorbed.

Efforts must be made to prevent a rise in IOP during induction, surgery and extubation. Anaesthetics that raise IOP like ketamine may be avoided if possible. Anaesthesia should be maintained until reversal of neuromuscular blockade, return of spontaneous breathing and extubation. Use of a laryngeal mask (instead of tracheal intubation) as discussed above and a small dose of propofol (0.5 mg/kg) immediately prior to extubation are useful in preventing IOP rise and smoothening of the extubation process.

The surgery is not particularly painful and usual non-steroidal analgesic medications may be used. Opioids should be avoided as they are associated with adverse effects like respiratory depression and vomiting. A subtenon block and/or topical anaesthetic (lignocaine) are safe alternatives to intravenous fentanyl for perioperative analgesia [26]. Subtenon block also reduces the incidence of oculocardiac reflex (OCR) and the requirement of post-operative analgesia.

Position of the globe is an indicator of the depth of general anaesthesia [27]. When muscle relaxants are given during general anaesthesia, the extraocular muscles are the last striated muscles to relax. If the eye moves during the surgery, the surgeon should indicate to the anaesthetist to deepen the anaesthesia.

Although OCR is uncommon in cataract surgery and frequently associated with strabismus surgery, yet the anaesthetists should be vigilant for it, especially in patients with trauma. It is typically recognized by sinus bradycardia associated with traction on extraocular muscles (typically medial rectus) or pressure on globe and immediately reverts on removal of the stimulus [28]. The use of atropine (20 μg/kg) at induction reduces its occurrence. It is interesting to note that children who develop an OCR during surgery are more likely to have post-operative nausea and vomiting. Hence, preventing the OCR reduces the incidence of post-operative vomiting [29].

Post-operative apnoea is life threatening in infants and the recovery team should be watchful for it [30].

5.5.3 Examination Under Anaesthesia

Examination under anaesthesia (EUA) of both eyes should be performed in all patients prior to draping. The examination should include handheld slit lamp examination, keratometry, retinoscopy, indirect ophthalmoscopy, measurements of axial length, intraocular pressure and corneal diameters. These provide an opportunity to detect often missed findings and achieve greater accuracy in biometry in an otherwise uncooperative child.

A surgical time out to reconfirm the details of the patient, the eye and the procedure should be an essential step prior to draping. There can be no greater misfortune than to operate on the incorrect patient or the wrong eye.

5.6 Surgical Steps

5.6.1 Instrumentation and Draping

Besides the instruments used in all cataract procedures, age-appropriate speculum, sutures for closure of incision, viscocohesive ophthalmic viscosurgical device

Table 5.1 Pediatric cataract trolley

Speculum
Collibri forceps
McPherson forceps
Suture tying forceps
Utrata/intraocular forceps
Vanna's scissors
Needle holder
Sinsky hook
Iris repositor/spatula
Simcoe irrigation-aspiration two way cannula
Hydrodissection cannula
Phacoaspiration hand piece
Cystotome
MVR knife
Keratome 2.8/3.0 mm
Trypan blue dye
OVDs (Cohesive e.g. 1.4% sodium hyaluronate and Dispersive e.g. 2% Hydroxypropyl methylcellulose)
Sutures (10-0 nylon and/or 10-0 vicryl)
Phacoemulsification and vitrectomy equipment should also be ready

(OVD) like 1.4% sodium hyaluronate, and instruments for anterior vitrectomy should be available in all pediatric cataract trolleys. The instruments used in pediatric cataract surgery are listed in Table 5.1 and Fig. 5.2.

Proper positioning of the head with an age-appropriate head ring and shoulder support should be ensured.

5.6.2 Incisions

(a) Paracentesis (Side port) incisions can be one or two depending on the technique of surgery followed by the surgeon. Two side port incisions about 180 degrees apart, one on each side of the planned main incision should be made, to provide a 360-degree reach. A sharp micro vitreoretinal (MVR) knife should be used to give a 0.9–1.2 mm width biplanar clear corneal incisions near the limbus (Figs. 5.3, 5.4 and 5.5). If the chamber becomes shallow at any step, injection of OVD should be done before proceeding.
Using an anterior chamber maintainer is an option that helps maintain constantly deep anterior chamber and reduces IOP fluctuations. It also maintains mydriasis and washes out any bleeding or pigment release that may inadvertently occur. It is introduced at 6 o'clock position at this stage. Infusion of balanced salt solution (BSS) containing adrenaline 1:500,000 is used during the surgery.

(b) The multiplanar (biplanar or triplanar) limbal main incision should be made with a 2.2, 2.8 or 3.0 mm keratome (depending on the width of the IOL cartridge). This incision should be valvular tunnel with the internal entry

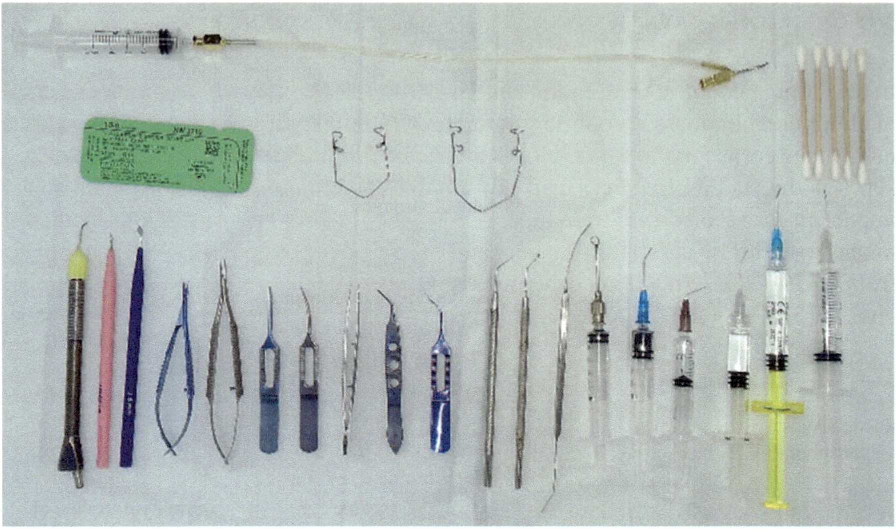

Fig. 5.2 Pediatric cataract trolley—Anticlockwise from bottom left: Irrigation aspiration handpiece, lancetip 0.9 mm (MVR may be substituted), keratome 2.2 mm, Vanna's scissor, needle holder (Castroviejo), suturing forceps (Castroviejo-straight and curved), forceps (Pierse Hoskins, McPherson lens holding, Utrata), Sinskey hook, posterior capsule polisher (Nightingale), iris repositor (Dastoor), irrigating wire vectis, trypan blue dye, cystotome, sodium hyaluronate, hydroxypropyl methylcellulose, 27G hydrodissection cannula on 2 ml syringe, sterile mop sticks (merocel sponge may be substituted), irrigation-aspiration cannula (Simcoe), wire speculums, 10-0 nylon suture

smaller (Figs. 5.3, 5.4 and 5.5). It should be made in the superior quadrant to ensure that it is protected by the eyelid. If implantation of IOL is not planned the surgery may be completed through the side ports using bimanual irrigation aspiration and anterior vitrectomy without the need for the main incision provided the CCC can be performed with a cystotome.

(c) If implantation of a non-foldable IOL is planned or even otherwise a sclerocorneal tunnel incision may be used. For this after conjunctival peritomy and use of minimal bipolar cautery a scleral scratch incision is made about 2 mm from the limbus. It is then dissected with a crescent blade as a 3.0–6.0 mm wide (depending on IOL size) sclerocorneal tunnel about 1–2 mm into clear cornea. The entry into the anterior chamber is made perpendicular to the tunnel plane by making the keratome vertical and may be delayed till the time of implantation of IOL. It has been shown that the induced astigmatism is similar in both corneal and scleral tunnel incisions [31].

5.6.3 Anterior Capsulorhexis

Performing a CCC in children is more challenging than in adults due to elasticity of the capsule and frequent collapse of the anterior chamber. The prerequisites for

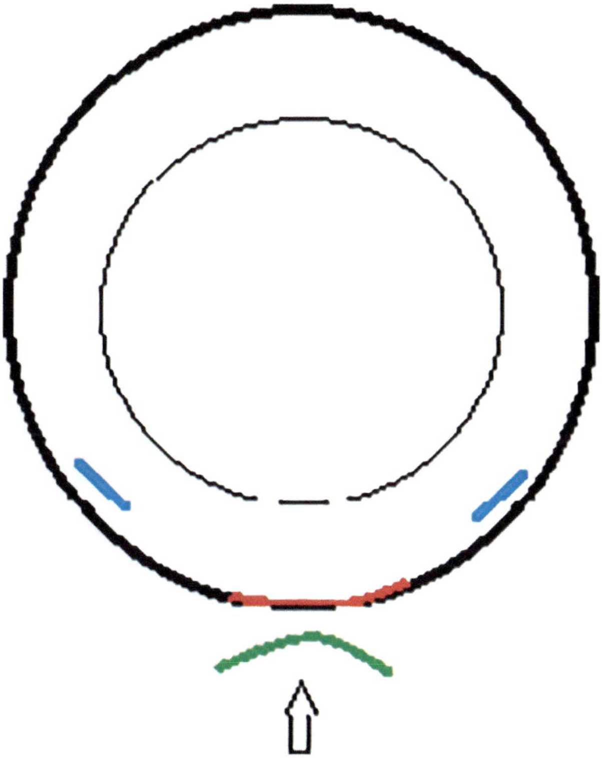

Fig. 5.3 A diagrammatic representation of the incision sites. The outer circle represents the limbus and the inner circle represents the dilated pupil. The surgeon sits superiorly (arrow). Blue lines are the position of side port (paracentesis) incisions, the red line is the site of limbal main incision and green line represents the outer lip of sclerocorneal tunnel

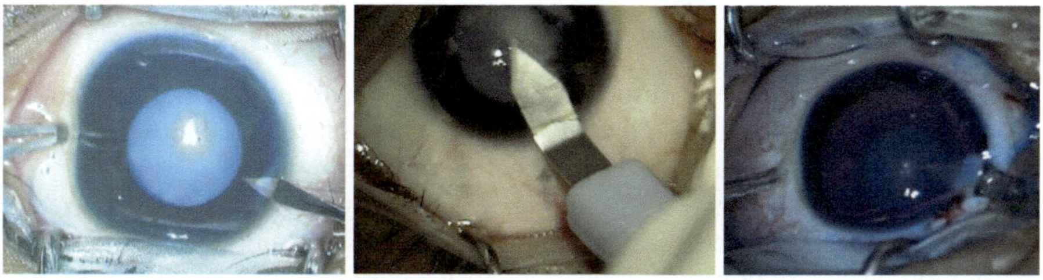

Fig. 5.4 Limbal incisions: Biplanar side-port incision (left), biplanar main incision with the blade remaining almost parallel to corneal surface during entry into anterior chamber (central), triplanar main incision with the blade dipping down at entry (right)

achieving success are mydriasis, good visibility, deep anterior chamber and appropriate instruments.

Preoperative atropinization should be done for mydriasis and cycloplegia. If pupil dilatation is inadequate it should be supplemented with preservative-free adrenaline (1:100,000) intraoperatively. Synechiolysis may be required if inflammation has occurred earlier. It should be performed in deep anterior chamber with minimal manipulation.

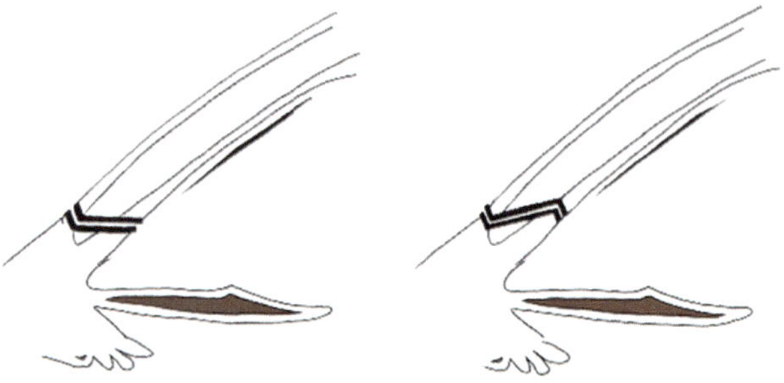

Fig. 5.5 Schematic drawings of biplanar and triplanar incision

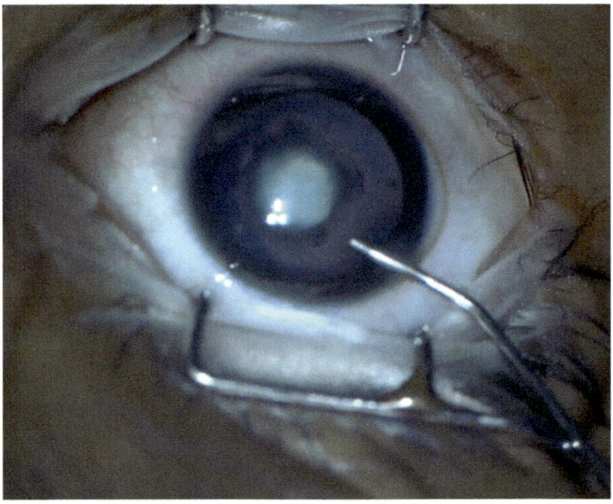

Fig. 5.6 The anterior chamber must be deepened with a cohesive OVD prior to initiation of CCC

Good visibility should be ensured by increasing the magnification and staining the anterior capsule with trypan blue dye (0.06%) in absence of red glow. The stain should be used under air and washed out before proceeding.

Higher viscosity cohesive OVDs like 1.4% sodium hyaluronate should be used to maintain a deep anterior chamber. Good side port incisions and delaying the main incision till necessary prevent chamber collapse. Overfill of the chamber should be achieved to make the anterior capsule concave anteriorly (Fig. 5.6) before proceeding with making a vertical nick with a cystotome.

Manual anti-clockwise CCC with an Utrata forceps introduced through the main incision remains the gold standard in children [32]. The capsule should be regrasped after each pull (Figs. 5.7 and 5.8). Inward pull should be maintained as the capsulorhexis in children tends to enlarge and run out. The advancing capsular flap should be kept flat. Should it become vertical or the chamber shallows, OVD should be reinjected. Lesser than 5 mm CCC should be made to cover the IOL optic all around. For beginners marking the size with an old trephine or using the newer microscope attachments may be useful to achieve greater accuracy [17].

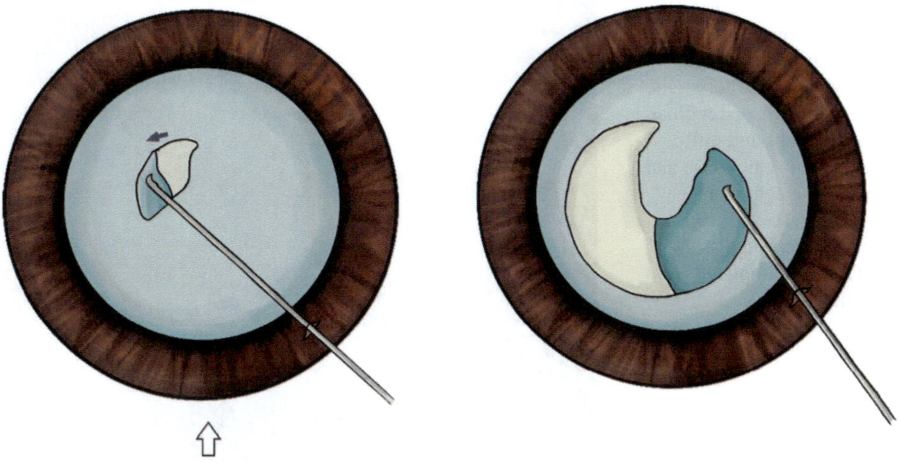

Fig. 5.7 Diagrammatic representation of CCC with cystotome. The position of the limbal entry is for a right-handed surgeon sitting superiorly (represented by the hollow arrow in the left figure). The initial nick is made about 6 clock hours away from the entry, flap flattened and direction of pull maintained anticlockwise and inwards (solid arrow). As the CCC proceeds (figure on the right) the flap is repeatedly flattened and reflected to represent the course of intended progression. The anterior chamber is kept deep during the entire procedure

While making the rhexis slightly smaller than the final size should be aimed as the opening stretches after completion.

Manual CCC with a cystotome or intra-vitreal forceps has the advantage of working through a smaller incision thus preventing chamber collapse, however, requires more skill. CCC may also be performed by vitrector, diathermy, plasma or radiofrequency probes but they are inferior in structure and strength compared to manual technique [33, 34]. A two incision push-pull technique for CCC may be tried as an alternative [35].

When an intumescent cataract is encountered, making a central puncture in the capsule with a sharp needle and aspirating the liquefied cortex reduces the intralenticular pressure. OVD is used to reform the anterior chamber and smaller than usual CCC is attempted as chances of 'run out' are high. The CCC may be enlarged later during surgery, if required.

Experience and patience enable successful completion of this difficult and important step of pediatric cataract surgery. It must be remembered that any discontinuity of capsular rim can easily extend to the equator due to increased capsular elasticity. The size, shape and integrity of the anterior capsulotomy are important for the long-term centration of IOL. Capsulotomy tears that extend to the posterior capsule may cause greater complications.

Some useful suggestions for successful pediatric cataract surgery have been listed in Table 5.2.

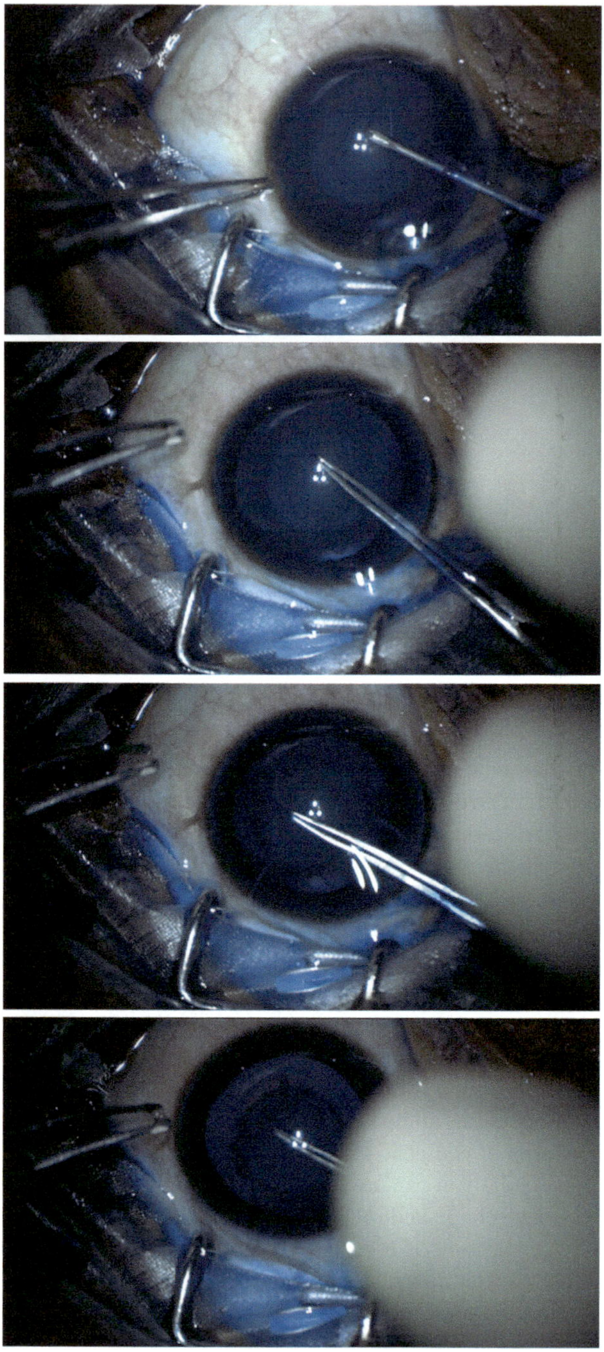

Fig. 5.8 Performing CCC (top to bottom): Initial nick in the anterior capsule is made with a cystotome, the flap is then grasped with an Utrata forceps and pull directed anti-clockwise and towards the centre. The proceeding flap is regrasped repeatedly and the CCC is completed from outside to within

Table 5.2 Pearls for pediatric cataract surgery

Incisions
• Biplanar or triplanar
• Suture closure
Capsulorhexis (CCC)
• Cohesive OVD
• Cystotome for puncture
• Utrata forceps for completion
• Frequent regrasping
• Aim smaller size
Posterior CCC
• Cohesive OVD
• Central, 3–3.5 mm diameter
• Use cystotome/Utrata forceps as for Anterior CCC
• Use vitrector if extension is threatening
Anterior vitrectomy (AV)
• Up to anterior third of vitreous removed
• Peaking and restricted movement of capsular rim suggests incomplete AV
Optic capture
• The IOL optic should be captured in PCCC to reduce visual axis opacification

5.6.4 Hydrodissection and Lens Aspiration

Hydrodissection of the cortical matter should be done in all quadrants using balanced salt solution in a 2-ml disposable syringe with a 27-G cannula under the margin of the CCC. Frequently with proper hydration the cortical matter flows out without the need for aspiration. Cortical cleaving hydrodissection in multiple quadrants not only eases the removal of lens matter but also enables the elimination of lens epithelial cells [36]. Hydrodissection should be avoided in posterior polar cataracts or those associated with posterior lenticonus.

Bimanual compared to coaxial irrigation and aspiration allows better chamber stability and 360 degrees reach. Meticulous cortical clean up at the equator and polishing the posterior capsule reduces the early VAO.

Occasionally hard nuclear matter may be encountered requiring the use of phacoemulsification for aspiration. Similarly, tough fibrotic plaques as seen in persistent fetal vasculature (PFV) may require excision with intraocular scissors.

Some surgeons prefer to perform lensectomy with the vitrectomy instruments through limbal incision with the advantage of not having to change instruments for posterior capsulotomy, secondary membranes or anterior vitrectomy.

The pars plana approach for the removal of crystalline lens has been discussed below.

5.6.5 Posterior Capsule Management

As discussed earlier VAO is the commonest late complication. Primary posterior continuous curvilinear capsulorhexis (PCCC) and anterior vitrectomy (AV) are effective in reducing and delaying it [37]. PCCC with AV should be performed in children below 4 to 6 years of age and in older children who are likely to be uncooperative for YAG laser capsulotomy (e.g. with mental illness and nystagmus) [38–42]. PCCC without AV may be performed in older children [35].

PCCC may be performed with an Utrata or intraocular forceps (Fig. 5.9). It is technically more challenging than anterior CCC (ACCC) as the posterior capsule is thinner (than anterior) with absence of support (offered by the crystalline lens during ACCC). The bag should be underfilled by viscocohesive OVD and vertical nick given with a cystotome inserted through the side port incision. A small amount of the viscoelastic may be carefully placed through the central puncture to push back the vitreous face, not allowing the flap to advance posteriorly [33]. Gentle pull and frequent regrasps of the advancing capsular edge will allow the creation of a 3–3.5 mm diameter central round PCCC, ideally, about 1–1.5 mm smaller than diameter of IOL optic [37]. Staining the posterior capsule with trypan blue dye in the absence of fundal glow and using the vitrectomy cutter to enlarge the capsular opening may be useful for beginners. It should, however, be kept in mind that the margins of opening created by vitrector are more prone to extending compared

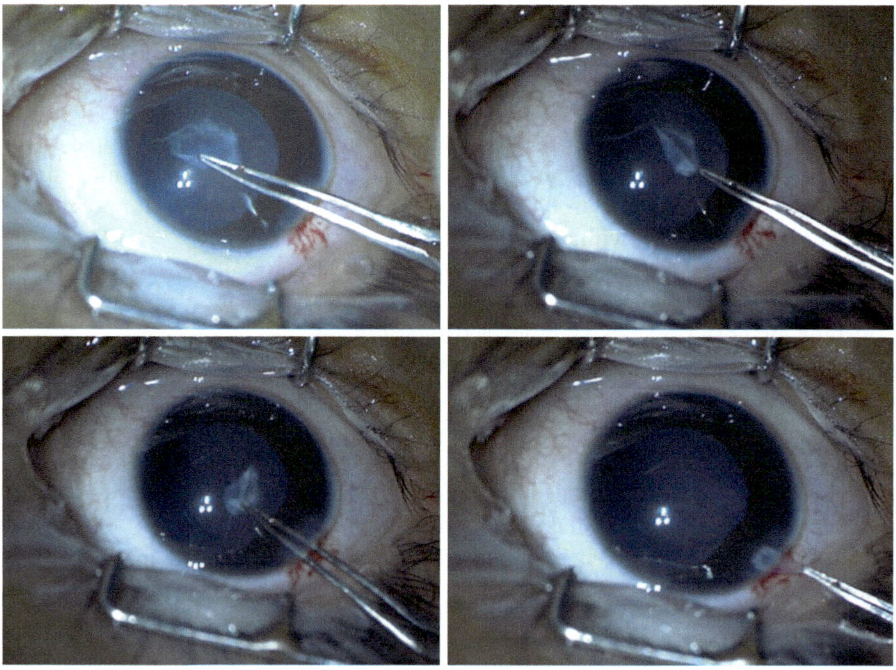

Fig. 5.9 Primary posterior capsulorhexis in an opaque posterior capsule with Utrata forceps

to those made manually, especially in infants where the capsule is more elastic [43–45]. A venturi pump system may be preferred over peristaltic pump for fibrotic capsules and membranes.

Posterior capsulotomy with anterior vitrectomy has also been described after implantation of the IOL and may be a safer alternative for beginners [46]. This is performed with the vitrectomy cutter, which is carefully manipulated behind the IOL. The common practice is to perform PCCC before IOL implantation if the limbal approach is being used. However, if the pars plana approach is being used, the posterior capsulectomy and vitrectomy are generally performed after IOL implantation as discussed in the next section [37].

5.6.6 Anterior Vitrectomy

Anterior vitrectomy in children besides reducing the formation of VAO, allows easier placement of IOL in the bag, reduces complications like pupillary capture of IOL and secondary glaucoma [47]. Generous anterior vitrectomy also markedly reduces the immediate postoperative iritis [48–50]. A 23 or 25 G handpiece should be inserted through one paracentesis incision with irrigation port through the other. Preferred parameters are cutting rate of 400–800 cuts/min and flow rate of about 30 ml/min and 300–400 cc vacuum. Central anterior vitrectomy up to 2 mm depth and 360 degrees under the margins of the PCCC is done taking care not to damage the margin by keeping the vitrectomy port directed posteriorly [32, 33]. Movement and curling back of the PCCC margin indicate completion. When in doubt, a minimal quantity of diluted triamcinolone acetate may be used to stain the vitreous.

Posterior capsulectomy and anterior vitrectomy may also be done through the pars plana after IOL implantation and closure of the main anterior incision. This approach a useful modification from purely limbal approach described earlier and pars plana approach discussed in the next section. Irrigation is maintained through the anterior infusion and a conjunctival opening followed by sclerotomy made with a microvitreoretinal (MVR) blade 2.5–3.0 mm posterior to limbus. This provides adequate access to the posterior capsule and allows wide anterior vitrectomy.

5.6.7 Pars Plana Vitrectomy with Lensectomy

Primary surgery by pars plana approach is preferred by some surgeons, in infants, when IOL implantation has not been planned. The advocates of this technique list reduced incidence of vitreous prolapse, wider reach, lesser damage to corneal endothelium and iris tissue as its advantages [51–53]. It also makes the second surgery easier. Two sclerotomies (one in the superonasal quadrant and the other in the superotemporal quadrant) as described above are made at pars plana. Balanced salt solution infusion containing epinephrine (1 in 500,000) is introduced through one sclerotomy. Through the other a 23 gauge or 25 gauge vitrectomy handpiece is used to perform anterior vitrectomy, posterior capsulotomy (sparing 2–3 mm peripheral rim of the posterior capsule) and lensectomy. A rim of the anterior capsule is also left untouched. Lesser postoperative inflammation is reported with the pars plana approach [54].

A useful tip is to turn off the infusion before withdrawal of the vitrectomy cutter from the eye to avoid incarceration of vitreous in the sclerotomy wound, which may cause complications later. Disadvantages of this approach are the need for additional skills, possibility of vitreous incarceration, loss of integrity of capsular bag, difficulty in visualization with inadequate mydriasis, risk of retinal dialysis and ciliary body detachment.

Weighing the pros and cons, the pars plana approach should be limited to eyes with comorbid conditions like microcornea and microphthalmos, in expert hands [55].

5.6.8 IOL Implantation

The choice of IOLs has been discussed in an earlier chapter. The ideal IOL would be the one with hydrophilic anterior surface and hydrophobic posterior surface [37]. Preferred are hydrophobic acrylic or heparin surface-modified hydrophilic foldable IOLs for implantation into the capsular bag [9, 56, 57]. For sulcus implantation a three piece lens with prolene haptics is preferred as it causes lesser pigment release and inflammation over prolonged periods [58, 59].

For implantation of the IOL the capsular rim (bag with anterior and posterior CCC) is inflated with OVD and the main incision enlarged to 2.8 mm. The foldable IOL is inserted gently so that the leading haptic pushes against the back surface of the anterior CCC and as it goes behind the anterior CCC the injector is slightly withdrawn and pushed down to lift the nozzle (cartridge) within the eye anteriorly (towards the cornea). This enables the trailing haptic to get released in the sulcus or anterior chamber and prevents the leading haptic from proceeding through the PCCC. The trailing haptic is then carefully dialled into the bag (Fig. 5.10).

Implanting a non-foldable IOL (in indications like traumatic capsular bag instability) is done through a pre-constructed larger incision (sclerocorneal tunnel). After the leading haptic is placed in the capsular bag the trailing haptic is dialled in.

5.6.9 Optic Capture

'Optic Capture' is a technique described to ensure long-term stability of the IOL when either anterior or posterior CCC is not intact or larger than desirable thereby potentially destabilizing the IOL [60]. The CCC being used for capture should be intact and smaller than the size of the optic. The procedure is performed after suturing of the main incision but before removal of the viscoelastic. It is best done with a rigid (non-foldable) or a foldable three piece IOL [61]. This procedure places the optic closer to the nodal point when the haptics are placed in the sulcus and the optic is engaged (captured) by the anterior CCC into the capsular bag [62, 63]. With haptics in

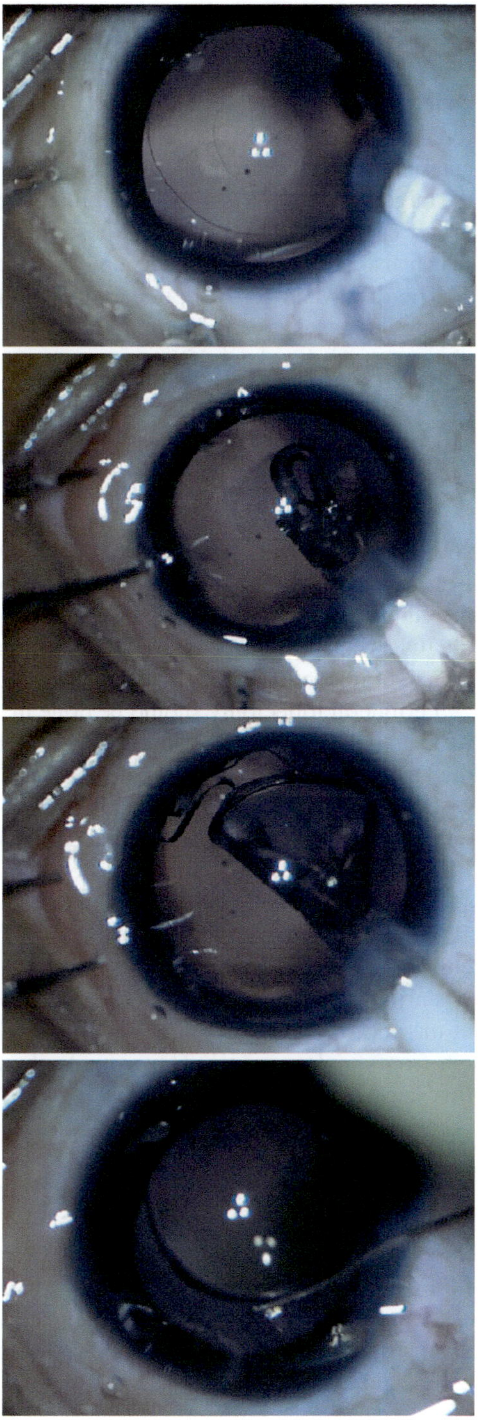

Fig. 5.10 Injection of IOL (top to bottom): The anterior and posterior CCC are focussed, IOL injection started and as the leading haptic goes behind the anterior capsule the injector is slightly withdrawn and pushed down to allow the release of the trailing haptic in anterior chamber, which is then dialled into the bag

the bag, capturing the optic with posterior CCC is done [64]. The latter is also called posterior capture of the IOL, and should be attempted only when the margins of the PCCC are intact and at least 1.5 mm smaller than the optic (Fig. 4.2). This frequently done procedure helps in maintaining a clear visual axis and also reduces the need for subsequent visual axis clearing procedures as it enables 360-degree apposition of anterior and posterior capsule rims except for the haptic–optic junctions. This reduces the migration of proliferating lens epithelial cells into the visual axis. The obliteration of space between the anterior and posterior capsules ensures tight fixation of the IOL which also prevents anterior movement of vitreous [10].

The disadvantages of optic capture are that it is technically challenging and it makes IOL exchange difficult should it be required later. However, it allows the placement of piggyback IOLs to correct refractive errors.

5.6.10 Viscoelastic Aspiration, Peripheral Iridectomy and Incision Closure

A thorough removal of the viscoelastics should be done from all quadrants and even from behind the IOL by gently tapping on it or negotiating the aspiration probe from the edge of the optic. However, a small amount of viscoelastic may be left behind the IOL when posterior capture of the IOL has been done [33]. Viscocohesive OVDs come out in continuity but dispersives are removed in parts.

Peripheral iridectomy should be done in eyes left aphakic. It may also be done in patients with uveitis and trauma. A vitrectomy cutter is used and it is performed as the last step before the closure of incision.

Decreased scleral rigidity, high likelihood of rubbing eyes and difficulty in post-operative examination warrants meticulous securing of all incisions in children. Limbal or sclerocorneal main incisions are sutured with 10-0 nylon, 9-0 vicryl or 10-0 vicryl [65]. Paracentesis (side port) incisions should be secured with a single 10-0 nylon suture in children below 2 years of age and maybe left unsutured in older children if they maintain their integrity after hydration. It is always safer to suture when in doubt. We prefer to leave a bubble of sterile air in the anterior chamber at the end of the surgery along with 0.1 ml of preservative free 0.5% moxifloxacin from single-use vial. The wounds should be rechecked for water tightness at this stage.

5.6.11 Subconjunctival/Subtenon Injections

Subconjunctival injection containing 0.2 ml (40 mg/ml) gentamicin, and 0.1 ml (4 mg/ml) dexamethasone is routinely given.

A subconjunctival or subtenon injection of triamcinolone acetonide may be given in patients where significant post-operative inflammation is expected (e.g. associated uveitis) [7].

5.6.12 Post-operative Medications

Post-operatively eyes are bandaged for 24 hours. When the bandage is opened, 0.3% gatifloxacin (or 0.5% moxifloxacin) and 1% prednisolone acetate 6 times a day (t/d) with 1% cyclopentolate 2 t/d eye drops are recommended for 4 weeks. Difluprednate 0.05% 4 t/d is an alternative to prednisolone acetate 1% and homatropine 2% can be used instead of cyclopentolate 1% [66]. The children may also be given oral amoxicillin (40 mg/kg/day) + clavulanic acid (10 mg/kg/day) in divided doses for 1 day preoperatively and 4 days after surgery prophylactically.

Oral prednisolone 1–1.5 mg/kg for 3 days preoperatively and 2 weeks postoperatively with 1 week taper may be given when exaggerated inflammatory response is expected as in uveitic cataracts [6]. Another option to overcome early postoperative inflammation in these patients is a single per operative dose of intravenous methylprednisolone 5–10 mg/kg.

It should be kept in mind that in pediatric eyes the peak inflammatory reaction may appear on the second or third day. Moreover, the symptoms may be deceiving. Hence, it is important that the children are examined post-operatively every day for 3 days. The topical steroids should be tapered over 6–8 weeks. After discharge on the fourth day, the children are examined every week for 1 month and then at 3–6 month intervals.

5.7 Common Per-operative Complications and Their Management

Incisions may become uniplanar making them prone to leakage and iris prolapse. If iris prolapse is troublesome it may be wise to close the defective incision with sutures and carefully make a new one. However, if surgery can be completed through the original incision, one may proceed with caution and suture it at completion.

Anterior capsule is prone to stretching and beginners often have an extension of the CCC into the periphery. One should aim for a smaller than planned opening from the beginning. If the CCC runs out at one end it is wiser to start afresh at the other end and attempt completion by connecting it to the part that has extended. It may be possible to achieve an eccentric but appropriate-sized opening with some patience. If this is not possible it is advisable to do a small-sized can opener capsulotomy with multiple small nicks, to avoid any long tags of the capsule. The edges of the opening may be rounded after IOL implantation. In the absence of good anterior CCC it is important to achieve an appropriately sized posterior CCC and perform posterior optic capture to ensure IOL stability.

Should an inadvertent posterior capsular tear/rupture (PCR) occur, its extension should be prevented by not allowing sudden changes in IOP, as is done in adults. Irrigation pressure should be lowered and sudden withdrawal of instruments avoided. Dispersive OVD should be placed over the tear and careful completion of cortical aspiration done. With some experience and patience, it is possible to convert the PCR into a circular posterior CCC. If manual conversion appears difficult, it may be done with a vitrector. IOL implantation in the bag should not be attempted in an incomplete posterior CCC, which is prone to extension. It is advisable to implant a three-piece IOL in the sulcus and perform its optic capture in anterior CCC in this case.

While injecting a foldable IOL it is common for the leading haptic to advance into the sulcus instead of the bag. In this situation, the trailing haptic should be allowed to open in the anterior chamber and the leading haptic manipulated into the bag with an IOL dialler. Once its position is confirmed, the trailing haptic may be dialled into position. If the entire IOL is in the sulcus after unfolding, one of the haptics should be nudged out into the anterior chamber before attempting to reposition into the bag. In the bag positioning of the IOL is confirmed by observing the margins of anterior and posterior CCC, above and below the IOL, respectively.

If one is careless while injecting or if the IOL unfolds with a jerk, it is possible that the leading haptic unfolds behind the posterior capsular into the vitreous. Further injection should be halted and the injector withdrawn to allow the trailing haptic to unfold in the anterior chamber. The trailing haptic should then be used to withdraw the IOL and carefully manipulate the leading haptic into the capsular bag. Injecting OVD behind the IOL is helpful. Should the entire IOL be noticed behind the posterior capsule at any stage, it is wise to seek help from a vitreoretinal surgeon rather than proceeding blindly.

5.8 Considerations in Concurrent Ocular Comorbidities

5.8.1 Microphthalmos

Microphthalmos is often associated with rubella cataracts (Fig. 5.11). Small eyes pose an additional challenge in management, but maybe the only hope of providing any useful vision in these children. Preoperative intravenous mannitol, clear corneal

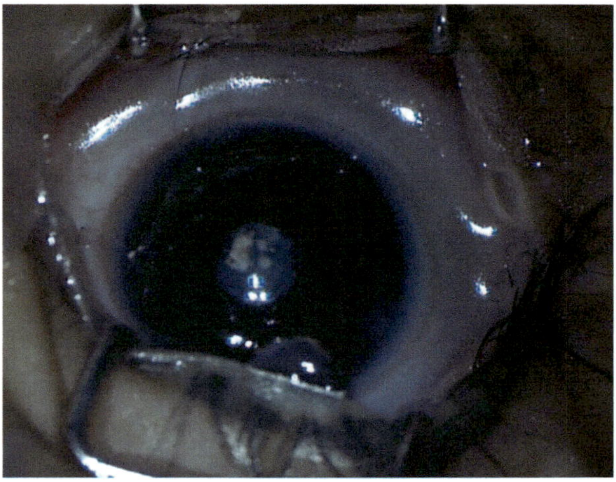

Fig. 5.11 Per operative photograph of a microphthalmic eye with dense nuclear cataract

incisions and generous use of viscoelastics are helpful. There is an increased likelihood of posterior capsular tear for which the surgeon should be vigilant. All incisions should be secured at the end of surgery. These eyes are best left aphakic in the primary surgery. Approaching the cataract through the pars plana may be a better option as has been discussed earlier. Postoperatively aphakic correction should be given and retina examination performed. Customized smaller-sized IOLs may be considered at about 2–3 years of age. Implanting an IOL too large for the eye is fraught with complications of which glaucoma is the commonest.

5.8.2 Lenticonus

Lenticonus is localized bulging of the capsule of the lens along with its underlying cortex. The diameter of the bulge is between 2 and 7 mm. The bulge may occur anteriorly or posteriorly. The anterior bulge has to be differentiated from lentiglobus in which protrusion involves the entire surface (Fig. 3.13).

Posterior lenticonus is commoner, usually unilateral and presents in children [67, 68]. It should be suspected in eyes with unilateral cataract localized to the central posterior capsule and adjacent subcapsular cortex. Intraoperative care should be taken as congenital weakness of the posterior capsule may occur [69]. Hydrodissection should be avoided.

Anterior lenticonus is rare, associated with Alport syndrome, usually bilateral and presents in adults [70].

5.8.3 Lens Coloboma/Subluxated and Dislocated Cataract

While dealing with zonular insufficiency associated with cataract, it is important to assess the area of involvement in terms of clock hours and the cause of the defect to determine whether the condition is progressive.

In progressive conditions like Marfan syndrome, initially the child should be managed with refractive correction as has been discussed elsewhere and later when there is a risk of dislocation of the crystalline lens, lensectomy should be considered. In non-progressive conditions like trauma or coloboma, the management depends on the severity of zonulodialysis. Up to 3 clock hours of zonular damage does not require any additional intraoperative step, except being careful to avoid sudden changes in IOP to prevent extension of dialysis (Fig. 5.12). A three piece IOL should be implanted in the bag with the haptics oriented in the axis of the zonulodialysis. Manipulation of the IOL once it is in the bag should be minimal. Any vitreous prolapse would require vitrectomy. When the zonular damage is between 3 and 6 clock hours (Fig. 7.8), implantation of an endocapsular ring should be done prior to IOL implantation, provided the posterior capsule is intact. When the zonulodialysis is more than 180 degrees, sutured ring segments would be required. These manoeuvres are challenging and should be undertaken in children only by experts.

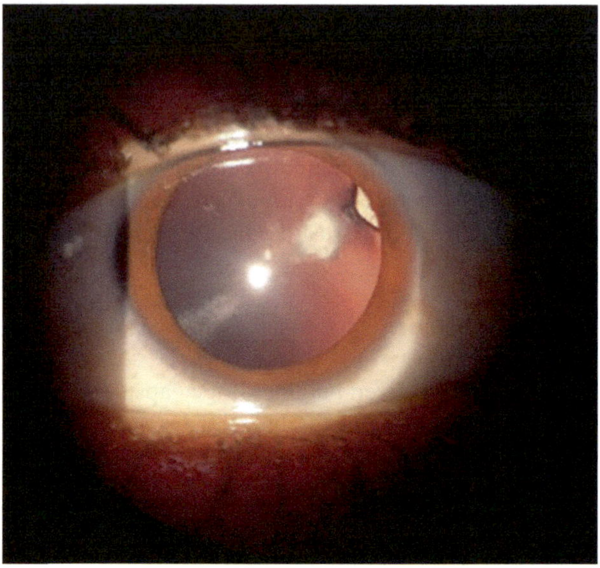

Fig. 5.12 Small subluxations up to 3 clock hours do not require an additional procedure

In eyes with anterior dislocation of crystalline lens, intralenticular aspiration and peripheral iridectomy with or without anterior vitrectomy are indicated [71]. Posterior dislocation is best managed by a vitreoretinal surgeon. Lensectomy with anterior chamber supported, iris and scleral fixated IOLs are alternatives in large subluxations and dislocations where bag or sulcus implantation is not possible [72]. Management of subluxated cataract has also been discussed in Chap. 7.

5.8.4 Buphthalmos

Cataract surgery in buphthalmic eyes presents unique challenges with IOL power calculation, compromised corneal endothelium, large capsular bag and stretched sclera. Special endothelium protective OVDs like *Viscoat* (Alcon Surgical Inc.) having sodium hyaluronate and chondroitin sulphate as contents may be used. Sulcus implantation with capturing of optic in anterior capsulorhexis and bag implantation without primary posterior capsulorhexis have been suggested as modifications to avoid post-operative decentration of the IOL [73, 74].

5.8.5 Persistent Fetal Vasculature

The pathogenesis and spectrum of PFV have been discussed in Chaps. 1 and 2. Intraoperative bleeding from the hyaloid artery remnants is a common complication during posterior capsulotomy and anterior vitrectomy. Endocautery of the blood vessels is required to stop bleeding. Fugo plasma blade has been used for posterior capsulotomy with a successful outcome in florid anterior PFV [75]. While anterior

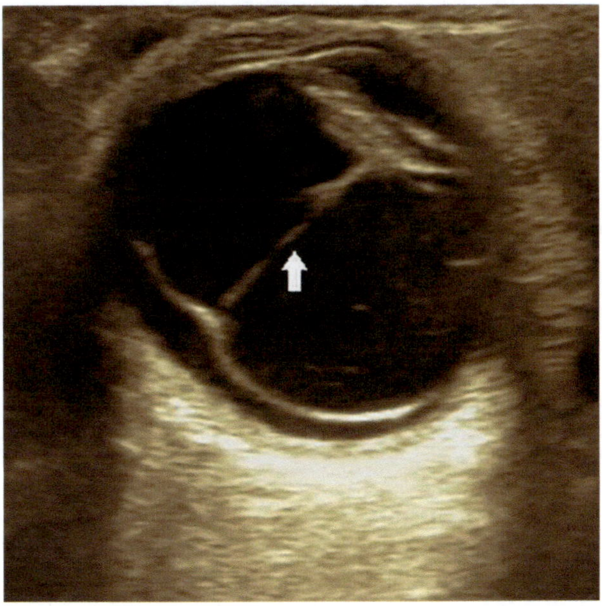

Fig. 5.13 B scan showing persistent fetal vasculature (arrow) (Image courtesy: Dr. Neha Agarwal, Lucknow, India)

PFV has a reasonable prognosis with appropriate management, the prognosis of posterior PFV is usually poor. It is associated with retinal detachment, retinal dysplasia and optic nerve dysmorphism [39] (Fig. 5.13).

5.8.6 Uveitis

Pediatric cataract associated with uveitis presents several challenges like intraocular inflammation, presence of synechiae, small pupil and difficulty in performing CCC. Juvenile idiopathic arthritis (JIA) is the commonest cause of uveitis and secondary cataract in children [5]. Intraocular inflammation should be controlled medically for at least 3 months prior to cataract surgery. While elimination of flare may be impossible in long-standing inflammation, absence of cells in anterior chamber and vitreous should be ensured. Topical and oral corticosteroids may be given preoperatively, as discussed earlier. Releasing fibrous bands on the pupil by gentle manoeuvres with forceps and carefully pulling the pupillary margin with two hooks placed 180 degrees apart to release posterior synechiae enables dilation (Fig. 5.14). Further, synechiolysis can usually be done with viscodissection or a spatula. Pupil expansion devices like iris hooks may be required if these manoeuvres fail. Pigment on anterior capsule tends to impede or divert the CCC and should be removed by viscopolishing or by irrigation and aspiration before initiating the CCC. We prefer to leave children with JIA aphakic as inflammation often flares up after IOL implantation. A small, peripheral iridectomy should be done to overcome the possibility of postoperative iris bombe. Postoperatively local, topical and systemic steroids along with cycloplegics are given as discussed earlier.

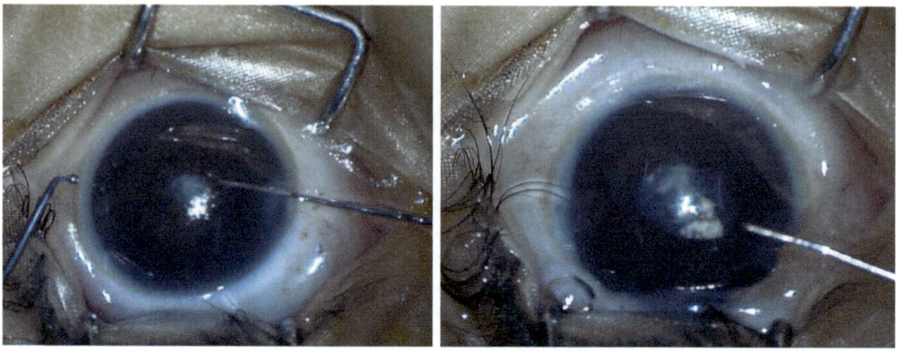

Fig. 5.14 Per operative photographs showing a miotic pupil with posterior synechiae (left) and after synechiolysis (right)

5.9 Prognosis

Developmental cataract has better prognosis than congenital cataract [76]. Congenital cataract also has good prognosis with timely diagnosis and surgery before 6 weeks of age. Delayed presentation, unilaterality, presence of strabismus, nystagmus, ocular or systemic morbidities and irregular postoperative follow ups are associated with poorer prognosis [18, 77].

5.10 Summary

- The anatomical and physiological differences from an adult eye make several surgical steps different in a pediatric eye.
- Surgery is performed under general anaesthesia. The pediatric anaesthetists are an integral part of the team and have to cater to special requirements of intraocular surgery.
- In pediatric eyes the incisions require suturing, continuous curvilinear capsulorhexis is difficult, the space in anterior chamber limited and posterior capsule requires special management. These eyes are also more prone to inflammation.
- Primary posterior capsulorhexis and anterior vitrectomy are crucial steps to ensure long-term media clarity.
- Learning skills like lensectomy, posterior capsulorhexis, optic capture and using vitrector for membranectomy/capsulotomies are essential for a pediatric cataract surgeon.
- Intraoperative complications are due to break in attention, impatience, improper instruments or lack of experience. For surgeons, it is advisable to first be well versed with adult cataract surgery and then perform the initial pediatric cataract procedures under supervision.
- Extra vigilance is required in the post-operative period for early detection of complications.

Acknowledgements The authors acknowledge the support of Mr. Ritwik Srivastava for designing the diagrams of this chapter.

Multiple Choice Questions

1. Which is the best option regarding management of congenital cataract?
   (a) Bilateral cataracts should be operated at an earlier age compared to unilateral.
   (b) Intraocular lens implantation may be deferred in bilateral cataract operated in early infancy.
   (c) Paracentesis incisions may be left suture less in infants.
   (d) Posterior capsulorhexis is technically easier than anterior capsulorhexis.

   Answer: *b. Intraocular lens implantation may be deferred in bilateral cataract operated in early infancy.* Unilateral cataract warrants urgent surgery for fear of dense amblyopia. Intraocular lenses may be implanted as a secondary procedure in children operated in early infancy. All incisions should be sutured in infants. Crystalline lens offers support and anterior capsule is thicker than posterior making it technically easier.

2. Which of the following are true with regards to visual axis opacification (VAO) in children:
   (a) VAO occurs due to improperly done surgery and its chances are minimal after a good surgery.
   (b) Posterior capsulorhexis and anterior vitrectomy almost eliminates the possibility of VAO in infants.
   (c) Posterior capsule may be left intact in children above 5–6 years of age as the chances of its opacification are minimal.
   (d) VAO management may require repeated procedures.

   Answer: *d. VAO management may require repeated procedures.* VAO occurs even after good surgery in children as the lens epithelial cells are rapidly dividing. Intraoperative measures only reduce and delay its occurrence. The posterior capsule is left intact in older children as they are cooperative for laser capsulotomy later. VAO management may require multiple procedures as the opacification may recur.

3. Which of the following is true with regards to anaesthesia in pediatric cataract surgery:
   (a) Surgery under local anaesthesia may be considered in older children with traumatic cataract.
   (b) Laryngeal mask is not recommended for intraocular surgeries.
   (c) Liberal use of local phenylephrine is safe to achieve mydriasis.
   (d) Coughing during extubation may cause a significant increase in intraocular pressure.

   Answer: *d. Coughing during extubation may cause a significant increase in intraocular pressure.* Coughing during extubation causes increase in IOP which may cause an improperly secured wound to open. General anaesthesia should be preferred in presence of trauma due to unpredictability of the surgery. Moreover, the use of peribulbar block significantly raises the IOP making the intraocular contents prone to prolapse. Laryngeal mask is preferred as it does not cause coughing during removal. Phenylephrine may cause a sudden rise in blood pressure and should be used cautiously in children.

4. All of the following make pediatric cataract surgery more challenging than adults *except*:
   (a) Compact vitreous gel
   (b) Increased capsular elasticity
   (c) Decreased scleral rigidity
   (d) Lesser space in capsular bag

   Answer: *a. Compact vitreous gel.* Solidified vitreous gel prevents vitreous from prolapsing easily during surgery and reduces the incidence of post-operative cystoid macular oedema. Capsular elasticity makes capsulorhexis difficult. Reduced scleral rigidity prevents incisions from being self-sealing. Lesser space in capsular bag makes in the bag IOL implantation difficult.

5. In case there is an inadvertent posterior capsule tear which of the following is *not* a standard management option:
   (a) Attempting to convert the tear into a circular posterior capsulorhexis.
   (b) Implanting a three-piece IOL in sulcus with optic capture.
   (c) Implanting a single-piece IOL in sulcus with optic capture.
   (d) Implanting a single piece foldable IOL in bag after posterior capsulorhexis.

   Answer: *c. Implanting a single-piece IOL in sulcus with optic capture.* The posterior capsule tear should be converted into a posterior capsulorhexis and usual hydrophobic acrylic single-piece IOL implanted into the bag. If conversion to capsulorhexis fails, a three-piece IOL (rigid or foldable) should be implanted in the sulcus and its optic capture attempted in anterior capsulorhexis. A single-piece IOL should not be implanted in the sulcus as it causes inflammation and pigment release.

Annexure 1: Consent for Pediatric Cataract Surgery

Name of Child **Parents Name**

Age/ Sex **Medical Record Number** **Date**

Address

Phone Number

A.1 Introduction

This information is given to you so that you can make an informed decision about the eye surgery of your child. Before you sign the INFORMED CONSENT DOCUMENT you have the right to ask any questions you might have about the operation.

Cataract means opacity in the natural lens of the eye. Cataract formation may occur in children at any age and may even be present at birth. It affects about 3 out of 10,000 children. It may affect one or both the eyes and has a variety of causes like maternal infections during pregnancy, genetic abnormalities and trauma. In many cases, the cause remains unknown. Surgery is done if the cataract is visually significant and does not allow normal visual development. This decision is best made by your ophthalmologist. Once it has been decided that the child requires surgery, it should not be delayed to enable the child to have a normal visual development. This is in contrast to cataracts in adults where delay in surgery does not affect the visual outcome.

The surgery is performed under general anaesthesia and involves removal of the cataractous lens and implantation of an artificial intraocular lens (IOL) in its place. In older children, this may be done in a single sitting, however, in very young children or those with some other complication the IOL implantation may be done in a second surgery. This decision is also best made by your ophthalmologist. If the cataract is present in both eyes, surgery if the second eye will be done within a few days or weeks of the first eye after the first eye starts recovering.

A.2 Post-operative Care

The operated eye of the child will be bandaged/covered for 24 hours after surgery. When the cover is removed the eye may be swollen, red and painful for a few days after the surgery. The child will be given oral medication and eye drops post-operatively for a few weeks. It is essential that the parents ensure that the instructions regarding the medication and hygiene are followed carefully. The child must not rub his/her eyes. The medications may be required for a prolonged period in certain cases for maximal benefit. The children will be required to come for follow ups initially every day for a few days, then every week and subsequently at monthly and three monthly intervals. Some of the follow ups may even require examination under general anaesthesia. The parents must understand that the surgery is only the start of treatment and the children will require lifelong care of eyes. Role of the parents will be as important as the ophthalmologist in ensuring a satisfactory visual outcome. The children will need glasses which will keep changing as the child grows. If your child has any associated systemic or ocular abnormality, he/she may require additional investigations/referrals/surgery for same.

A.3 Post-operative Course and Possible Complications

Cataract surgery performed by the experienced team is generally very safe. However, no surgical procedure is without risks. Risks related to General Anaesthesia have been mentioned in a separate document which you are expected to sign. The ocular risks of pediatric cataract surgery include but are not limited to the following:

1. Posterior capsular opacification (PCO) is the commonest cause of decreased vision after surgery. With the latest developments in techniques and equipment, its occurrence has reduced but it can occur in all children, especially younger ones. Management of this condition may require additional surgery under general anaesthesia or a laser procedure depending on the age of the child.
2. The child will need to wear glasses after surgery and frequent change of glasses will occur as the child grows. The parents must understand that the IOL implanted has a fixed power and as the child's eye grows the changing power is compensated for by glasses. It is of paramount importance that the children wear appropriate glasses or contact lenses as prescribed. Prescription of glasses will require repeated check-ups and may even require sedation/anaesthesia in uncooperative children.
3. Amblyopia (lazy eye) is a common cause of suboptimal visual outcomes after a successful surgery. The amblyopia is severe in prolonged duration of cataract, younger age of the child and in unilateral cataract. It is managed by appropriate glasses and occlusion therapy, compliance of which is to be ensured by the parents. This treatment may be required to continue for months or years after surgery.
4. Glaucoma (raised intraocular pressure) is a cause of delayed visual loss after a successful surgery. It is commoner in eyes with associated comorbidity. To monitor its development and treat it timely the ophthalmologist may measure the intraocular pressure of the eyes at follow ups. The parents must ensure that scheduled follow up visits are not missed.

5. Retinal detachment is a rare but potentially sight-threatening sequelae. It may happen days, months or years later and requires surgery for treatment.
6. Intraocular infection leading to endophthalmitis or panophthalmitis is extremely rare but may be sight and eye threatening. It may require urgent management in the form of injections or surgery.
7. Strabismus (Squint) and nystagmus (involuntary oscillations of eye/s) may be present initially or occur later and require separate management.
8. The results of any surgery cannot be guaranteed.

It is important that you commit to regular long-term follow ups and adherence to prescribed treatment for satisfactory surgical outcome. Timely post-operative visits will help the medical team in adequate assessment of child, detection and timely management of the conditions above, should they occur.

A.4 Patient Consent (to Be Signed by Legal Guardian in Children)

The advantages and disadvantages, risks and possible complications of the present surgery and alternative treatments have been explained to me by my ophthalmologist. There may arise unwanted emergency situations during surgery. In that situation, I give my full authority to my treating doctor to take any necessary decision for my patient's wellbeing. Although it is impossible for the doctor to inform me about every possible complication that may occur, the doctor has answered all my questions to my satisfaction. In signing this informed valid consent for operation. I am stating that I have been offered a copy of this consent.

I have informed the doctor and personnel of all known allergies, medications being taken and previous eye as well as medical conditions. I understand that I have responsibilities in relation to my child's healthcare and eye care. I understand what my child should and should not be doing before and after the procedure. I have received instructions and agree to follow them.

Further, I consent to the observing, using medical record, photographing or televising of the procedure to be performed for medical, scientific, research, education purpose and publication in scientific journals provided my identity is not revealed by the picture or by descriptive text accompanying them.

I hereby give permission to release/publish medical data and/or video/audio record/photograph the current medical procedure and the procedures performed in subsequent/follow up visits for the advancement of medical knowledge.

I have read and understood the consent form, and all my queries have been answered, and I authorize my surgeon to proceed with the operation on my child's............(right or left) eye.

Signature and Thumb Impression of Patient/Legal Guardian ………………….
Patient Name: ………………………………………………………..
Guardian's Name ………………………… Relation with patient …………..
Address …………………………………………………………………
Phone No.: ……………. Date …………… Place …………………………..

Witness 1 **Witness 2**

Signature:
Name:
Address:
Phone:

Declaration by Doctor

I, Dr. ....declare that I have explained the nature and consequences of the procedure to be performed, and discussed the risks that particularly concern the patient.

I have given the patient an opportunity to ask questions and I have answered these.

Doctor's signature
Date: ……………………………………………….. Place: ……………………

Witness 1 **Witness 2**

Signature:
Name:
Address:
Phone:

Annexure 2: Checklist for Receiving a Pediatric Cataract Patient in the Operating Room

Confirm identity and procedure

- Medical record number
- Patient name & Guardian's name
- Procedure mentioned
- Eye marked and confirmed with records

Consent

- Consent for surgery
- Consent for general anaesthesia
- Consent for multiple surgery/poor prognosis in patients with trauma

Medical history/workup

- Allergies
- Medical and treatment history
- Bscan / Ocular Imaging available
- Systemic workup

- Pre-anaesthetic clearance
- Pediatrician clearance

Pre-operative orders/Availability of implant

- Nil orally since
- Pre operative instructions of Pediatrician & Anaethetist followed
- Topical/systemic antibiotic prophylaxis
- Intravenous mannitol (if advised)
- IOL power calculation
- IOL available
- Refraction of other eye available (if pseudophakic)
- Pupil dilated

References

1. Bell CM, Hatch WV, Cernat G, Urbach DR. Surgeon volumes and selected patient outcomes in cataract surgery: a population-based analysis. Ophthalmology. 2007;114(3):405–10.
2. Gimbel H, Dubbar J. Pediatric cataract surgery. In: Albert D, Miller J, editors. Principles and practice of ophthalmology. 3rd ed. St. Louis, MO: Saunders; 2008. p. 1479–85.
3. Zetterström C. Intraocular lens implantation in the pediatric eye. J Cataract Refract surg. 1997;23:559–600.
4. Ronneburger A, Basarab J, Howland HC. Growth of the cornea from infancy to adolescence. Ophthalmic Physiol Opt. 2006;26:80–7.
5. Krag S, Olsen T, Andreassen TT. Biomechanical characteristics of the human anterior lens capsule in relation to age. Invest Ophthalmol Vis Sci. 1997;38:357–63.
6. Raizman MB. Chapter 57: Prolonged intraocular inflammation. In: Steinert R, editor. Cataract surgery. 3rd ed. Irvine, CA: Saunders Elsevier; 2010. p. 687–94.
7. Khokhar SK, Pillay G, Dhull C, Agarwal E, Mahabir M, Aggarwal P. Pediatric cataract. Indian J Ophthalmol. 2017;65(12):1340–9.
8. Hiles DA. Intraocular lens implantation in children with monocular cataracts 1974-1983. Ophthalmology. 1984;91:1231–7.
9. Hemo Y, BenEzra D. Traumatic cataracts in young children. Correction of aphakia by intraocular lens implantation. Ophthalmic Pediatr Genet. 1987;8:2032–207.
10. Gimbel H, Debroff BM, Dunbar JA, Nihalani BR. Chapter 26: Surgical management of pediatric cataracts and aphakia. In: Steinert R, editor. Cataract surgery. 3rd ed. Irvine, CA: Saunders Elsevier; 2010. p. 311–32.
11. Basti S, Aasuri M, Reddy MK, et al. Heparin surface modified intraocular lenses in pediatric cataract surgery: prospective randomised study. J Cataract Refract Surg. 1999;25:782–7.
12. Klais CM, Hattenbach L, Steinkamp GWK, et al. Intraocular recombinant tissue-plasminogen activator fibrinolysis of fibrin formation after cataract surgery in children. J Cataract Refract Surg. 1999;25:357–62.
13. Zetterström C, Lundvall A, Kugelberg M. Cataracts in children. J Cataract Refract Surg. 2005;31(4):824–40.
14. Birch EE, Stager DR. The critical period for surgical treatment of dense congenital unilateral cataract. Invest Ophthalmol Vis Sci. 1996;37(8):1532–8.
15. Birch EE, Cheng C, Stager DR Jr, Weakley DR Jr, Stager DR Sr. The critical period for surgical treatment of dense congenital bilateral cataracts. J AAPOS. 2009;13(1):67–71.
16. Nallasamy S, Davidson SL, Kuhn I, Mills MD, Forbes BJ, Stricker PA, et al. Simultaneous bilateral intraocular surgery in children. J AAPOS. 2010;14:15–9.
17. Binder AP. Intra-operative OCT devices for ophthalmic use: an overview. Spectr Ophthalmol. 2014;28:2–5. http://www.springer.com/medicine/ophthalmology/journal/717

18. Sukhija J, Ram J. Pediatric traumatic cataract: maximizing the surgical outcome. J Cataract Refract Surg. 2012;38:2210–1.
19. Rabiah PK, Smith SD, Awad AH, Al-garni A, Al-mesfer SA, Al-turkmani S, et al. Results of surgery for bilateral cataract associated with sensory nystagmus in children. Am J Ophthalmol. 2002;134:586–91.
20. Chawla B, et al. Informed consent in ophthalmic surgeries. All India Ophthalmological Society. 2019.
21. Abdel M, Mahdy S. Effect of flurbiprofen and dexamethasone acetate in prevention of surgically induced miosis during cataract surgery. J Am Sci. 2011;7:474–8.
22. Agrawal S, Singh V, Vinod Kumar BM, Meena M, Srivastava RM, Katiyar V. Immediate sequential bilateral cataract surgery in children in a government medical university in India. J Clin Ophthalmol Res. 2020;8:14–7.
23. Goswami D, Seetharamaiah S, Kedia SK, Nayak BK, Akshat S. Anesthetic dilemma in planning bilateral cataract surgery for an infant associated with congenital cardiac anomaly. Indian J Ophthalmol. 2015;63(6):548–9.
24. Engelhardt T, Johnston G, Kumar MM. Comparison of cuffed, uncuffed tracheal tubes and laryngeal mask airways in low flow pressure controlled ventilation in children. Pediatr Anaesth. 2006;16:140–3.
25. Gulati M, Mohta M, Ahuja S, Gupta VP. Comparison of laryngeal mask airway with tracheal tube for ophthalmic surgery in paediatric patients. Anaesth Int Care. 2004;32:383–9.
26. Ghai B, Ram J, Makkar JK, Wig J, Kaushik S. Subtenon block compared to intravenous fentanyl for perioperative analgesia in pediatric cataract surgery. Anesth Analg. 2009;108:1132–8.
27. Dahan E, Salmenson BD. Pseudophakia in children: precautions, technique, and feasibility. J Cataract Refract Surg. 1990;16(1):75–82.
28. Blanc VF, Hardy JF, Milot J, Jacob JL. The oculocardiac reflex: a graphic and statistical analysis in infants and children. Can Anaesth Soc J. 1983;30:360–9.
29. Allen LE, Sudesh S, Sandramouli S, Cooper G, McFarlane D, Willshaw HE. The association between the oculocardiac reflex and postoperative vomiting in children undergoing strabismus surgery. Eye. 1998;12:193–6.
30. Welborn LG, Ramirez N, Oh TH, Ruttimann UE, Fink R, Guzzetta P, et al. Postanesthetic apnea and periodic breathing in infants. Anesthesiology. 1986;65:658–61.
31. Bar-Sela SM, Spierer A. Astigmatism outcomes of scleral tunnel and clear corneal incisions for congenital cataract surgery. Eye (Lond). 2006;20:1044–8.
32. Vasavada AR, Nihalani BR. Pediatric cataract surgery. Curr Opin Ophthalmol. 2006;17:54–61.
33. Grueterich M, Lackerbauer CA, Kampik A. Performance of the Acri. Smart 46S intraocular lens in pediatric microincision cataract surgery. J Cataract Refract Surg. 2008;34(4):591–5.
34. Wilson ME Jr. Anterior capsule management in pediatric cataract surgery. Trans Am Ophthalmol Soc. 2004;102:391–422.
35. Hamada S, Low S, Walters B, Nischal K. Five-year experience of the 2-incision push–pull technique for anterior and posterior capsulorrhexis in pediatric cataract surgery. Ophthalmology. 2006;113(8):1309–14.
36. Vasavada AR, Trivedi RH, Nihalani B. Multiquadrant hydrodissection. In: Wilson Jr ME, Trivedi RH, Pandey SK, editors. Pediatric cataract surgery; Techniques, complications, and management. Philadelphia, PA: Lippincott, Williams & Wilkins; 2005. p. 77–9.
37. Alexandrakis G, Peterseim MM, Wilson ME. Clinical outcomes of pars plana capsulotomy with anterior vitrectomy in pediatric cataract surgery. J Am Assoc Pediatr Ophthalmol Strabismus. 2002;6(3):163–7.
38. Batur M, Gül A, Seven E, Can E, Yaşar T. Posterior capsular opacification in preschool-and school-age patients after pediatric cataract surgery without posterior capsulotomy. Turk J Ophthalmol. 2016;46(5):205.
39. Chapter 23. Childhood cataracts and other pediatric lens disorders. Pediatric ophthalmology and strabismus. American Academy of Ophthalmology, 2015–2016. Vol. 6, p. 291–308.
40. Parks MM. Management of the posterior capsule in congenital cataracts. J Pediatr Ophthalmol Strabismus. 1984;21(3):114–7.

41. Buckley EG, Klombers LA, Seaber JH, Scalise-Gordy A, Minzter R. Management of the posterior capsule during pediatric intraocular lens implantation. Am J Ophthalmol. 1993;115(6):722–8.
42. Trivedi RH, Wilson ME. Posterior capsulotomy and anterior vitrectomy for the management of pediatric cataracts. In: Wilson Jr ME, Trivedi RH, Pandey SK, editors. Pediatric cataract surgery; Techniques, complications, and management. Philadelphia, PA: Lippincott, Williams & Wilkins; 2005. p. 83–92.
43. Wilson ME, Trivedi RH, Bartholomew LR, Pershing S. Comparison of anterior vitrectorhexis and continuous curvilinear capsulorhexis in pediatric cataract and intraocular lens implantation surgery. A 10-year analysis. J AAPOS. 2007;11:443–6.
44. Andreo LK, Wilson ME, Apple DJ. Elastic properties and scanning electron microscopic appearance of manual continuous curvilinear capsulorhexis and vitrectorhexis in an animal model of pediatric cataract. J Cataract Refract Surg. 1999;25:534–9.
45. Neuhann T. Capsulorrhexis. In: Steinert RF, editor. Cataract surgery—technique, complications, management. St. Louis, MO: Saunders; 2004. p. 137–45.
46. Kochgaway L, Biswas P, Paul A, Sinha S, Biswas R, Maity P, et al. Vitrectorhexis versus forceps posterior capsulorhexis in pediatric cataract surgery. Indian J Ophthalmol. 2013;61:361–4.
47. Mandal AK, Netland PA. Glaucoma in aphakia and pseudophakia after congenital cataract surgery. Indian J Ophthalmol. 2004;52(3):185.
48. Lambert SR, Drake AV. Infantile cataracts. Surv Ophthalmol. 1996;40:427–58.
49. Dahan E, Salmenson BD. Pseudophakia in children: precautions, techniques and feasibility. J Cataract Refract Surg. 1990;16:75–82.
50. Ahmadieh H, Javadi MA, Ahmadi M, et al. Primary capsulectomy, anterior vitrectomy, lensectomy, and posterior chamber lens implantation in children: limbal versus pars plana. J Cataract Refract Sirg. 1999;25:768–75.
51. BenEzra D, Rose L. The surgical approaches to pediatric cataract. Eur J Implant Refract Surg. 1990;2:241–4.
52. Cheah WM. A review of management of congenital cataract. Asia Pacific J Ophthalmol. 1989;1:22–6.
53. Green BF, Morin JD, Grant HP. Pars plana lensectomy/vitrectomy for developmental cataract extraction: surgical results. J Pediatr Ophthalmol Strabismus. 1990;27:229–32.
54. Dahan E. Pediatric cataract surgery. In: Yanoff M, Duker J, editors. Ophthalmology. 2nd ed. St Louis, MO: Mosby; 2004. p. 374–6.
55. Gimbel H, DeBroff B, Dunbar J, Nihalani B. Surgical management of pediatric cataracts and aphakia. In: Steinert R, editor. Cataract surgery. 3rd ed. Saunders Elsevier: Irvine, CA; 2010. p. 315–22.
56. Khokhar SK, Pillay G, Agarwal E, Mahabir M. Innovations in pediatric cataract surgery. Indian J Ophthalmol. 2017;65(3):210.
57. Basti S, Aasuri MK, Reddy MK, Preetam P, Reddy S, Gupta S, et al. Heparin-surface-modified intraocular lenses in pediatric cataract surgery: prospective randomized study. J Cataract Refract Surg. 1999;25:782–7.
58. Wilson ME, Apple DJ, Bluestein EC, Wang XH. Intraocular lenses for pediatric implantation: biomaterials, designs, and sizing. J Cataract Refract Surg. 1994;20(6):584–91.
59. Wilson ME, Bluestein EC, Wang XH. Current trends in the use of intraocular lenses in children. J Cataract Refract Surg. 1994;20(6):579–83.
60. Zhou HW, Zhou F. A Meta-analysis on the clinical efficacy and safety of optic capture in pediatric cataract surgery. Int J Ophthalmol. 2016;9(4):590–6.
61. Vasavada AR, Trivedi RH, Singh R. Necessity of vitrectomy when optic capture is performed in children older than 5 years. J Cataract Refract Surg. 2001;27(8):1185–93.
62. Faramarzi A, Javadi MA. Comparison of 2 techniques of intraocular lens implantation in pediatric cataract surgery. J Cataract Refract Surg. 2009;35(6):1040–5.
63. Xie YB, Ren MY, Wang Q, Wang LH. Intraocular lens optic capture in pediatric cataract surgery. Int J Ophthalmol. 2018;11(8):1403.
64. Gimbel HV, BM DB. Posterior capsulorhexis with optic capture: maintaining a clear visual axis after pediatric cataract surgery. J Cataract Refract Surg. 1994;20(6):658–64.

65. Lavrich JB, Goldberg DS, Nelson LB. Suture use in pediatric cataract surgery. A survey. Ophthalmic Surg. 1993;24:554–5.
66. Kaur S, Sukhija J. Difluprednate versus prednisolone acetate for inflammation following cataract surgery in pediatric patients: a randomized safety and efficacy study. Eye (Lond). 2017;31:506.
67. Cheng KP, Hiles DA, Biglan AW, Pettapiece MC. Management of posterior lenticonus. J Pediatr Ophthalmol Strabismus. 1991;28:143–9.
68. JS M, Schnall BM. Bilateral posterior lenticonus. Ophthalmic Surg. 1995;26:383–4.
69. Khalil M, Saheb N. Posterior lenticonus. Ophthalmology. 1984;91:1429–30, 43A.
70. Sonarkhan S, Ramappa M, Chaurasia S, Mulay K. Bilateral anterior lenticonus in a case of Alport syndrome: a clinical and histopathological correlation after successful clear lens extraction. BMJ Case Rep. 2014;2014:bcr2013202036.
71. Khokhar S, Aron N, Yadav N, Pillay G, Agarwal E. Modified technique of endocapsular lens aspiration for severely subluxated lenses. Eye (Lond). 2017;160
72. Kavitha V, Balasubramanian P, Heralgi MM. Iris-claw versus posterior chamber fixation intraocular lens implantation in pediatric traumatic cataract. Taiwan J Ophthalmol. 2016;6:69–74.
73. Sukhija J, Kaur S, Pandav SS, Kaushik S, Raj S, Ram J. Pediatric cataract surgery in buphthalmos. Eur J Ophthalmol. 2015;25(3):260–2.
74. Gupta PC, Singh RR, Pandav SS, Ram J. Rhexis fixation of intraocular lens in a case of buphthalmos with cataract. Nepal J Ophthalmol. 2016;8(15):71–3.
75. Sinha R, Bali SJ, Kumar C, et al. Results of cataract surgery and plasma ablation posterior capsulotomy in anterior persistent hyperplastic primary vitreous. Middle East Afr J Ophthalmol. 2013;20(3):217–20.
76. Gogate P, Patil S, Kulkarni A, Sahasrabudhe M, Shah M, Mahadik A, et al. Unilateral congenital and developmental cataracts in children in India: how useful were long-term outcomes of surgery? Miraj pediatric cataract study 4. Asia Pac J Ophthalmol (Phila). 2015;4:376–80.
77. Ram J, Gupta N, Sukhija JS, Chaudhary M, Verma N, Kumar S, et al. Outcome of cataract surgery with primary intraocular lens implantation in children. Br J Ophthalmol. 2011;95:1086–90.

Pediatric Cataract Surgery: Post-operative Complications and Their Management

6

Joyce J. Chan, Emily S. Wong, and Jason C. Yam

6.1 Introduction

Successful cataract surgery is only the first step on the long road of pediatric cataract management. Post-operative examination, refraction and measurement of intraocular pressure are often difficult due to limited cooperation. In some cases, sedation or examination under anaesthesia may be required. In addition, cataract surgery notoriously carries a higher risk of complications in infants and children than in adults. These include an intense post-operative inflammatory reaction and higher risks of wound leakage, visual axis opacification, refractive errors, secondary glaucoma and retinal detachment. Some eyes may also have other abnormalities that increase the risk of complications. As there is a lifelong risk of developing complications, children need to be followed long term. Most children will also require refractive correction and amblyopia treatment but compliance may be limited. Parental education is paramount, and a high level of vigilance and timely management of complications are essential to ensure good long-term outcomes (Table 6.1).

6.2 Early Post-operative Complications (within 4 weeks of surgery)

There is a higher risk of early post-operative complications following pediatric cataract surgery, but most of these can be prevented or minimized with optimized surgical techniques and careful perioperative management as has been discussed in earlier chapters.

J. J. Chan · E. S. Wong · J. C. Yam (✉)
Department of Ophthalmology and Visual Sciences, The Chinese University of Hong Kong, Hong Kong Eye Hospital, Kowloon, Hong Kong
e-mail: yamcheuksing@cuhk.edu.hk

S. Agrawal (ed.), *Pediatric Cataract*,
https://doi.org/10.1007/978-981-16-1736-2_6

Table 6.1 Common issues to be addressed after pediatric cataract surgery

• Difficulty in follow-up and examination; need for repeated sedation or examination under anaesthesia.
• Intense post-operative inflammatory reaction.
• Increased risk of wound leakage secondary to high tissue elasticity.
• Higher risk of visual axis opacification, secondary glaucoma and retinal detachment.
• Amblyopia management and visual rehabilitation.
• Parental education and ensuring long-term compliance.

6.2.1 Inflammation

Inflammation following cataract surgery is more intense in children than in adults. Factors that may further exacerbate inflammation include younger age, history of uveitis, intraoperative iris manipulation, prolonged surgery and sulcus rather than in-the-bag placement of the intraocular lens (IOL) [1]. In severe cases, inflammation may lead to fibrin formation, secondary membranes, pigment deposits on the IOL, posterior synechiae, secclusio pupillae and secondary angle closure glaucoma. Modern surgical techniques that limit iris manipulation and ensure capsular bag fixation of the IOL have resulted in less post-operative inflammation in young children.

6.2.1.1 Prevention: Pre-operative

Exaggerated post-operative inflammation is of particular concern in children with uveitic cataracts. Inflammation should be aggressively controlled before the surgery and the eye should ideally be quiescent for at least 3 months. A combination of topical and systemic steroids, immunosuppressive agents and biologics are often required, and the frequency of topical steroid and dosage of systemic steroids may need to be increased peri-operatively as prophylaxis. Control of inflammation should be achieved as soon as possible as any delay in surgery may increase the risk of deprivational amblyopia in young children. The decision to implant a primary intraocular lens for pediatric uveitic cataract remains controversial as has been discussed in earlier chapters [2]. IOL implantation may be considered only when uveitis has been controlled for about 3 months. In all children, pupil dilatation should be maximized pre-operatively with adequate use of mydriatic agents.

6.2.1.2 Prevention: Intraoperative

Intraoperatively, iris trauma and manipulation should be minimized. This can be achieved by careful wound construction to prevent iris prolapse, care when inserting and removing instruments through the wounds, appropriate use of viscoelastics, adequate pre-operative dilation and epinephrine added to the irrigation solution to reduce intraoperative miosis and floppy iris. An appropriately sized capsulorhexis and in-the-bag placement of IOL reduces post-operative iris chafing. Foldable hydrophobic acrylic IOL has been shown to produce less inflammation when compared with polymethyl methacrylate (PMMA) IOL in children [3]. At the end of the surgery, intracameral preservative-free or subconjunctival steroids are commonly employed. Heparin added into the intraocular irrigating solution to reduce fibrinous uveitis has also been reported [4]. Perioperative oral prednisolone and/or a bolus dose of intravenous steroid intraoperatively may be considered for uveitic cataracts.

6.2.1.3 Prevention: Post-operative

Post-operatively, topical steroids (e.g. prednisolone acetate 1% starting at every 1–2 h) are tapered over 4–12 weeks depending on clinical course. Steroid ointments can be used before bedtime but should be avoided during waking hours because of the possibility of blurred vision. In case of steroid response, a change to loteprednol or rimexolone is often helpful. Drop instillation is difficult in infants and young children, and parental compliance is paramount. In patients with a history of uveitis or in whom surgery is complicated, an exaggerated inflammatory response may be anticipated and the use of a short course of oral steroids (e.g. 1 mg/kg oral prednisolone for 1 week) may be considered. Some surgeons also prescribe cycloplegics post-operatively to reduce ciliary spasm, stabilize the blood–aqueous barrier, reduce the risk of synechia formation and dilate the pupil to facilitate examination, especially in infants. There is a risk of pupillary capture of the IOL if it is implanted in the ciliary sulcus, but the risk is minimal if the IOL is well positioned in the bag.

6.2.1.4 Management of Fibrinous Membranes

Despite the above measures, some infants and children still develop a severe fibrinous uveitis unresponsive to steroid therapy. The use of recombinant tissue plasminogen activator (rTPA) has been shown to be effective in removing a fibrinous membrane [5, 6]. However, if administered within 3 days of surgery there is a risk of inducing hyphaema. Other complications of rTPA include intraocular pressure elevation and band keratopathy. This treatment should be administered at institutes frequently handling pediatric cataract patients. Other options include simple mechanical and viscodissection of fibrinous membranes and synechiae. In some cases, Nd:YAG laser treatment may be helpful to clear the visual axis.

6.2.1.5 Toxic Anterior Segment Syndrome (TASS)

Toxic anterior segment syndrome (TASS) (Fig. 6.1), an acute severe post-operative intraocular inflammation that presents 12–24 h after cataract surgery, has also been reported in children [7, 8]. Features include diffuse corneal oedema, fibrin formation, sterile hypopyon and increased intraocular pressure. Most cases resolve with intense topical steroid treatment. However, permanent sequelae, including persistent corneal oedema, irregular pupil, peripheral anterior synechiae and glaucoma can develop in severe cases. TASS can be triggered by contamination or improper pH/osmolarity/ionic composition of various substances that gain entry into the eye during surgery. Adherence to proper protocols for cleaning and sterilization of intraocular surgical instruments is important to reduce the risk of TASS.

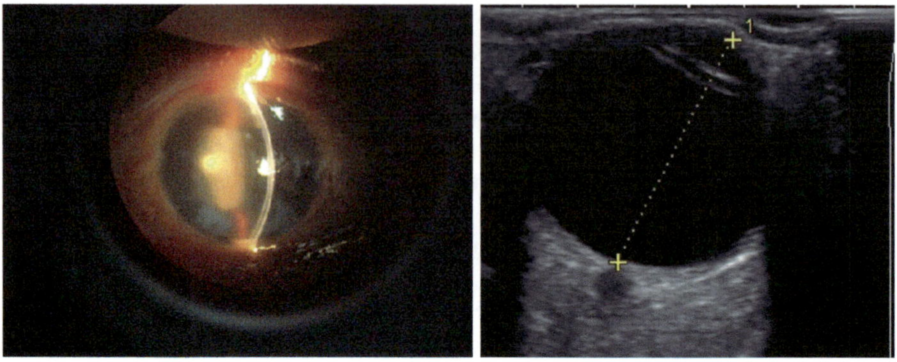

Fig. 6.1 Toxic anterior segment syndrome (TASS) is characterized by intense anterior segment inflammation, corneal oedema and raised intraocular pressure. However, unlike endophthalmitis there is lesser pain, the pupil dilates and the vitreous is anechoic on B scan. (Photo courtesy: Dr. Malvika Singh, Lucknow, India)

6.2.2 Endophthalmitis

Endophthalmitis is a rare complication after pediatric cataract surgery. Reported prevalence ranges from 0.07% to 0.45% [9, 10]. *Staphylococcus* and *Streptococcus* are the most common organisms identified. Risk factors include nasolacrimal duct obstruction and upper respiratory tract infection at the time of cataract extraction. Peri-operative topical antibiotics are frequently used for prophylaxis. Some surgeons administer subconjunctival or intracameral antibiotics. Loose non-absorbable sutures may become a nidus for infection and should be removed as soon as possible.

Post-operative endophthalmitis should be distinguished from intense inflammatory reaction or TASS. Endophthalmitis is typically more painful but this may be difficult to ascertain in infants or young children. The hallmark of endophthalmitis is vitritis and the vitreous should be clear in TASS (Fig. 6.2). Vitreous should be assessed on B Scan ultrasonography if media does not allow view on indirect ophthalmoscopy. Management for endophthalmitis in children is in principle the same as adults, which includes vitreous sampling, intravitreal antibiotics and vitrectomy.

The overall outcome is often poor, with over half of the patients having light perception or no light perception vision. Some reports have suggested that early vitrectomy may be associated with better visual outcomes [11, 12], but these retrospective reports also included post-traumatic cases and no randomized controlled trials are available.

Considering the risk of TASS and endophthalmitis, simultaneous cataract surgery in children with bilateral cataract is a debatable issue. In children with high risk due to general anaesthesia (GA), operating both eyes in single GA session appears a logical alternative. Furthermore, studies have shown that simultaneous bilateral cataract surgery offers advantages of expedited visual rehabilitation and

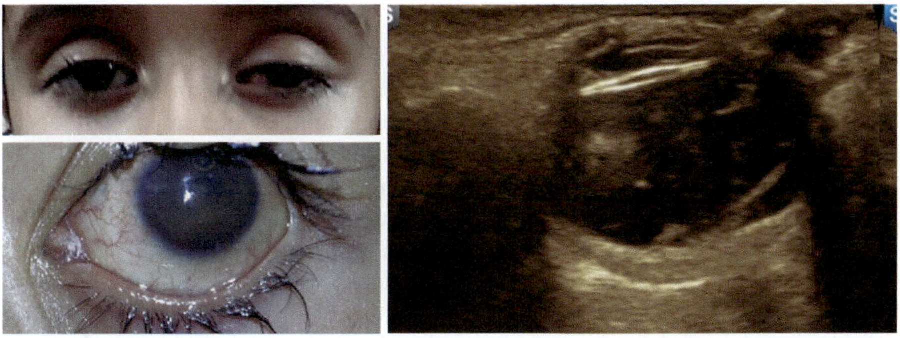

Fig. 6.2 Endophthalmitis should be suspected in presence of unexplained pain or crying in early post-operative period with lid oedema, circumcorneal congestion, exudates in anterior chamber, miotic pupil and vitreous exudates on B scan (B Scan image courtesy: Dr. Neha Agarwal, Lucknow, India)

reduced cost without any additional risk of complications like endophthalmitis [13, 14]. If bilateral simultaneous surgery is performed, it is important that the surgical team re-scrub and re-gown for each eye. The eyes should be individually prepped and draped, and a new set of instruments and solutions used for each eye. Should endophthalmitis be suspected a timely referral to a centre with vitreoretinal facilities can be sight saving.

6.2.3 Wound-Related Problems

Due to higher scleral and corneal elasticity in infants and children, wounds are not self-sealing and there is an elevated risk of post-operative wound leakage. Wounds should be carefully constructed and a sufficiently long tunnel is recommended. All corneal wounds should be sutured, preferably with absorbable sutures (e.g. 10-0 vicryl), and sutures may need to be more closely spaced to ensure watertight closure. Due to rapid wound healing, sutures tend to loosen earlier so they should be adequately tight when tied.

Loose sutures cause irritation, discomfort and may predispose to suture abscess and infection. If non-absorbable sutures are used, removal of loose sutures should be done at the slit-lamp, or under general anaesthesia in the operating room if there is limited cooperation.

A transparent shield may be used to prevent the young children from rubbing their eye in the early post-operative period. Wound leak may present as a shallow or flattened anterior chamber, a peaked pupil or incarceration of the iris in the wound. The chamber will need to be reformed, the iris repositioned and the wound re-sutured. Prompt repair is required to prevent infection, hypotony and permanent iris adhesions, which may lead to secondary glaucoma.

6.2.4 IOL-Related Complications

IOL-related complications such as pupillary capture, decentration or dislocation are more common in infants than in adults. These complications are more frequent when the IOL is placed in the ciliary sulcus or if the anterior capsulotomy is larger than the size of the IOL optic. Decentration can also occur due to asymmetric IOL fixation, traumatic zonular loss or inadequate capsular support. Late decentration is associated with excessive capsular fibrosis and posterior synechiae formation. Severe capsular phimosis with up to 15% shrinkage of capsular bag diameter, have been associated with smaller anterior capsulotomies [15]. A central circular anterior capsular opening of about 5 mm just covering the lens optic would be ideal to prevent decentration (Figs. 6.3 and 6.4).

Mild pupillary capture may be left untreated if it is not associated with decreased visual acuity or glaucoma but surgical release results in a rounder pupil and better IOL centration. In the early post-operative period, e.g. within the first month, the bag may be opened with viscoelastics and the IOL dialled back into place. Reverse capture of the optic of a sulcus-fixated IOL through the anterior capsulorhexis opening is also helpful. Otherwise, explantation of the IOL bag complex may be required in cases of significant IOL dislocation or decentration. Aphakia may then be corrected with spectacles or contact lenses. There is also the option of secondary scleral fixated IOL when the child is older. Evidence for sutured scleral fixated IOL in children is lacking and there is concern regarding suture breakage and IOL tilting as the eyeball grows with age. Some authors have reported early post-operative success with intrascleral haptic fixation in children, but no long-term data is available [16].

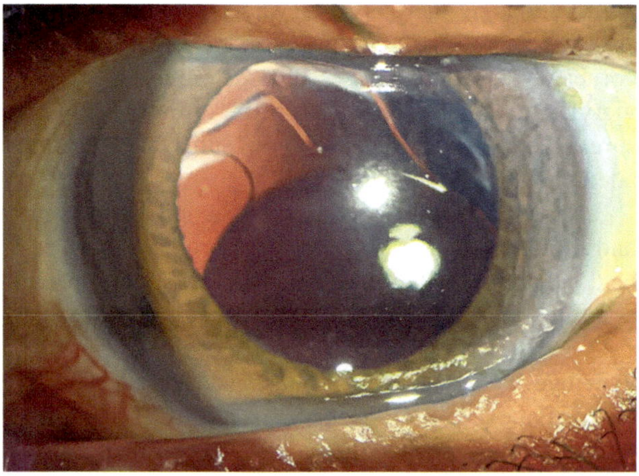

Fig. 6.3 Subluxated IOL in early post-operative period (Photo courtesy: Dr. Mohit Khattri, Kanpur, India)

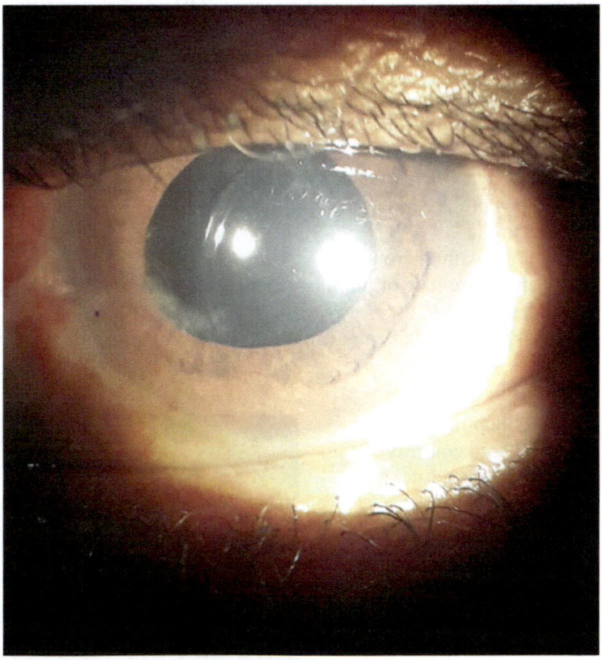

Fig. 6.4 Decentred IOL (Photo courtesy: Dr. Ankur Yadav, Lucknow, India)

6.2.5 Post-operative IOP Spike and Early-Onset Glaucoma

In the immediate post-operative period, IOP spikes can occur as a result of retained viscoelastics or lens matter, intense inflammation including TASS, hyphaema and vitreous prolapse into the angle. In addition, children are susceptible to steroid response, which tends to occur earlier and in a more marked fashion than in the adult population.

Early-onset glaucoma occurring in the first few months after pediatric cataract surgery is more likely to be due to angle closure than delayed-onset glaucoma, which is more commonly open-angle [17, 18] (Table 6.2). Angle closure glaucoma occurs most frequently in the early post-operative period in microphthalmic eyes secondary to pupil block. Pupil block can also result from IOL capture (Fig. 6.5) or secclusio pupillae and pupillary membranes due to intense inflammation. Intraocular pressure should be measured at each post-operative visit. This has been made easier with the availability of rebound tonometry, which allows IOP measurement in most infants and young children in the outpatient setting. Examination of corneal clarity, anterior chamber depth and the iris are also important.

The risk of post-operative IOP spike can be reduced by meticulous removal of viscoelastics, careful surgical technique to prevent iris trauma, adequate anterior

Table 6.2 Causes of early postoperative IOP rise

Open angle
• Steroid response
• Intense inflammation
• Retained viscoelastics or lens matter
• Hyphaema
• IOL related Uveitis-Glaucoma-Hyphaema syndrome
• Vitreous prolapse into angle
Closed angle
• Pupil block in microphthalmic eyes
• Secclusio pupillae or pupillary membranes due to intense inflammation
• IOL capture
• Aphakia without adequate anterior vitrectomy or patent peripheral iridectomy

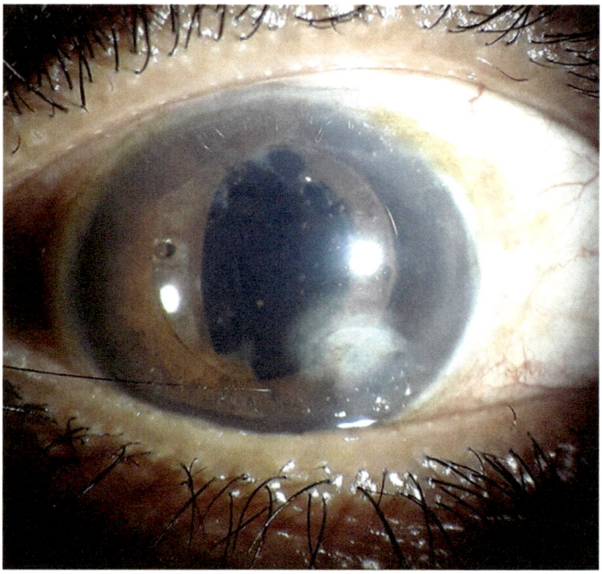

Fig. 6.5 Pupillary capture of IOL (Photo courtesy: Dr. Ankur Yadav, Lucknow, India)

vitrectomy and removal of vitreous from the anterior chamber (with the help of triamcinolone for visualization if necessary), and judicious use of peri-operative steroids to control inflammation while balancing the risk of steroid response. Post-operative IOP spikes can usually be managed with medical anti-glaucomatous therapy. For management of pupillary block, laser iridotomy can be attempted in older children, but surgical iridectomy and/or removal of membranes are required if laser iridotomy fails.

6.3 Late Post-operative Complications (after 4 weeks of surgery)

Complications of pediatric cataract surgery can occur months to years after the initial surgery, so long-term follow-up is important (Table 6.3). These late-onset complications can significantly affect visual rehabilitation. Timely management is paramount to achieve optimal long-term visual outcomes.

6.3.1 Visual Axis Opacification

Visual axis opacification (VAO) is rapid and nearly universal in infants and young children if the posterior capsule is left intact. It is caused by greater inflammation and proliferation of residual lens epithelial cells on the posterior capsule or anterior hyaloid face, and can lead to amblyopia if the visual axis is obscured (Fig. 6.6).

6.3.1.1 Prevention

The incidence of VAO is affected by the age of the patient, management of the posterior lens capsule and anterior vitrectomy, IOL design, material and site of fixation,

Table 6.3 Sample schedule for early post-operative follow-up (should be adjusted based on the patient's age and presence of complications)

Post-operative day 1 and 2
• Wound integrity (Seidel test if required), anterior chamber (depth and inflammation), red reflex, rebound (iCare) tonometry
Post-operative day 3
• Same as done on day 1 and 2
• Dilated fundal examination if possible
• Start spectacle wear (e.g. +20D temporary spectacles)
• Start patching in unilateral cases (e.g. 1 h/day for each month of life, maximum 6 h per day)
Post-operative week 1 (consider weekly follow-up for first month in infants or young children)
• Visual acuity, intraocular pressure, signs of endophthalmitis, post-operative inflammation, corneal clarity, wound and sutures, anterior or posterior iris synechiae, pupil shape, anterior chamber depth and reaction, IOL position, red reflex, dilated fundal examination
Post-operative month 1
• As above, post-operative inflammation should be minimal
• Refraction and start contact lens wear at post-op 3–4 weeks
Post-operative month 3, then visits every 3–6 months
• Visual acuity, compliance with patching/refractive correction, intraocular pressure, slit-lamp examination as above, ensure no significant visual axis opacification, refraction and dilated fundal examination (once every 6–12 months depending on age)

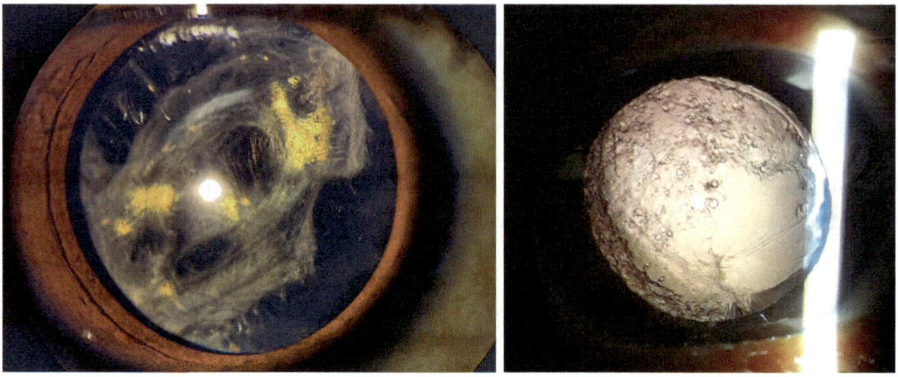

Fig. 6.6 Dense posterior capsular opacification in visual axis (Photo courtesy: Dr. Mohit Khattri, Kanpur, India)

the extent of cortical clean-up, surgical trauma and post-operative inflammatory response [19]. Straight-edged foldable acrylic lenses help prevent posterior capsular opacification in adult cataract surgery but are not sufficient in the pediatric population. Currently, primary posterior capsulotomy and anterior vitrectomy are performed routinely in infants and young children for prevention of VAO.

Removal of the posterior capsule in itself is not sufficient, as the anterior vitreous surface can serve as a scaffold for migration of lens epithelial cells. When primary posterior capsulotomy is not combined with anterior vitrectomy, the incidence of posterior capsule closure is up to 84% [17]. In infants whose posterior capsule had been retained, performance of a Nd:YAG capsulotomy was associated with high rate (57%) of recurrence of visual axis opacification across the anterior hyaloid face [20]. In contrast, reported rates of VAO after combined posterior capsulotomy and vitrectomy are lower and range from 0 to 27% [17]. A common practice is to perform manual posterior continuous curvilinear capsulorhexis and anterior vitrectomy with a limbal approach before IOL implantation. Some surgeons perform posterior capsulotomy and vitrectomy through a pars plana approach after in-the-bag placement of IOL. In a randomized controlled study of 45 eyes, no statistically significant difference in outcome measures was found between these two approaches [21].

Other techniques include optic capture through the posterior capsulorhexis with or without anterior vitrectomy as discussed in earlier chapters, and the bag-in-the-lens IOL implantation technique without anterior vitrectomy, in which the anterior and posterior capsules are fused with a specially designed IOL having a 360-degree groove around the IOL optic [22].

There is some minor variation in practice as to at what age the posterior capsule and anterior vitreous can be left intact, based on the risk of VAO and amblyopia, and whether the child will cooperate for laser capsulotomy at the slit-lamp. Some suggest primary posterior capsulotomy and anterior vitrectomy for all children under the age of 5 or 6 years [23, 24]. Vasavada et al. advise primary posterior capsulorhexis and vitrectomy for all children aged 0 to 3 years, primary posterior capsulorhexis only for children aged between 3 and 6 or 7 years, and an intact posterior capsule in children over the age of 6 to 7 years [17].

The authors perform primary posterior capsulotomy and anterior vitrectomy for all children who cannot tolerate laser capsulotomy at the slit-lamp, and this can be assessed pre-operatively by trying to insert a contact lens in the clinic. Children uncooperative for same are unlikely to allow laser post-operatively.

6.3.1.2 Management

When significant visual axis opacification develops, resulting in blurred fundal details or reduced visual acuity, early treatment is essential to reduce to risk of deprivational amblyopia. Before planning any surgical intervention for clearing the visual axis, posterior segment evaluation including assessment of lens-capsular bag complex should be done. Status of posterior capsule, extent of capsular fibrosis along with IOL position can be assessed using Ultrasound-biomicroscopy (UBM). Furthermore, the angle structures and capsular zonules can also be assessed using UBM before performing surgical membranectomy.

Neodymium-YAG Laser Capsulotomy

Nd:YAG laser is useful for performing secondary capsulotomies in older and cooperative children. In children who cannot cooperate with the procedure under topical anaesthesia, it can be performed under general anaesthesia using a specially mounted Nd:YAG laser for supine patients. If a conventional machine is used, the patient's head can be supported in the headrest in a lateral decubitus position (Figs. 6.7 and 6.8). In infants and younger children, the rate of VAO recurrence after Nd:YAG laser capsulotomy is high, as residual lens epithelial cells can still proliferative across the anterior hyaloid face. As secondary membranes are often thick and fibrous in young children, high energies may be required and there is a risk of IOL pitting (Fig. 6.9). Repeated treatments may be required.

Secondary Surgical Membranectomy

Secondary surgical membranectomy is required if Nd-YAG is unlikely to be effective, for example in younger children or in the presence of thick fibrous membranes or re-proliferation of cortical lens material. In the presence of an IOL, the procedure is done through the pars plana or pars plicata preferably. Limbal approach can be used in aphakic children and after tilting the IOL to insert the vitrector below it, in others.

6.3.2 Refractive Error

Appropriate optical correction after cataract extraction in infancy and childhood is critical to avoid ametropic and anisometropic amblyopia. Options include contact lens, spectacles and IOL implantation.

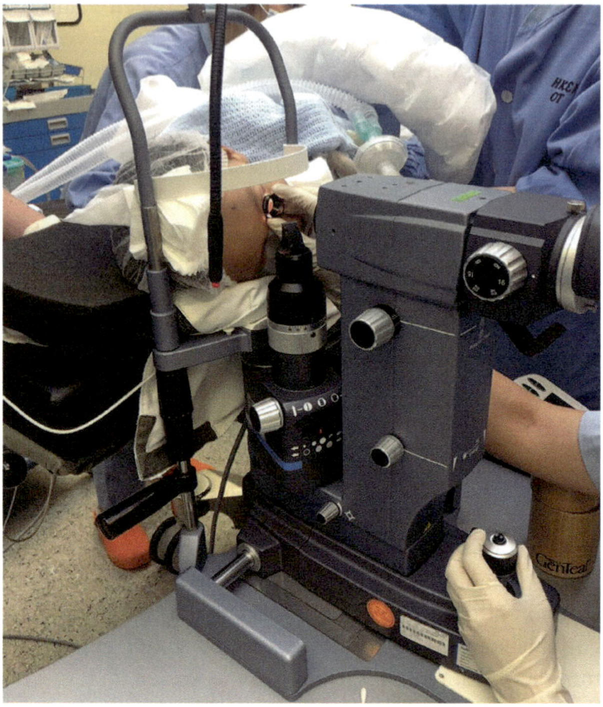

Fig. 6.7 Nd:Yag laser performed under general anaesthesia using a conventional machine, with the patient's head supported in the headrest in a lateral decubitus position

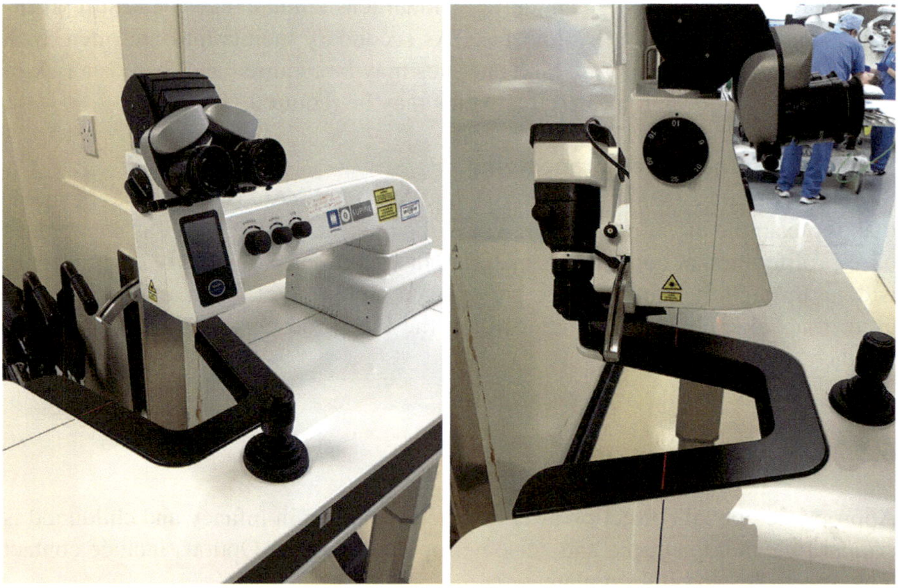

Fig. 6.8 Supine Nd:Yag machine enables easier capsulotomy under general anaesthesia

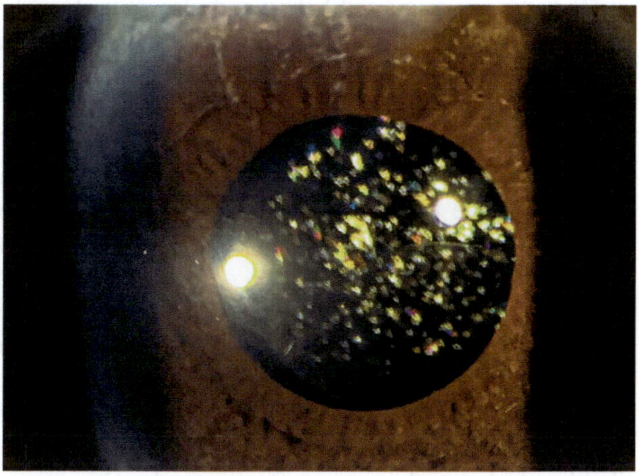

Fig. 6.9 Excessive pitting of IOL following careless Nd-YAG capsulotomy (Photo courtesy: Dr. Mohit Khattri, Kanpur, India)

6.3.2.1 Contact Lens and Spectacles for Aphakia

Contact lenses provide superior optical resolution, especially for unilateral aphakia. Motivated parents are needed, but compliance is usually good in infants. When the child reaches 2–3 years of age, parents may encounter more resistance and compliance may reduce. The authors usually perform pre-operative contact lens fitting to determine the base curvature and diameter, so that the appropriate contact lens can be ordered without delay once post-operative refraction is determined. Infants are usually overcorrected to leave them around −2 to −3 dioptres myopic to optimize near vision.

Spectacles are sometimes used for children with bilateral aphakia. However, high plus spectacles are associated with optical aberrations such as magnification, restricted visual field and pincushion distortion.

6.3.2.2 Primary IOL Implantation

Primary IOL implantation is now an accepted treatment in older children and performed increasingly in younger children and infants. IOLs more closely replicate the optics of the crystalline lens, ensure at least a partial optical correction at all times, and avoids the expense and compliance issues associated with contact lens. The Infant Aphakia Treatment Study (IATS) was a multi-centre randomized clinical trial that compared contact lens with IOL implantation in infants with a unilateral congenital cataract <7 months of age. After 5 years of follow-up, the study did not find a significant difference in visual acuity or incidence of glaucoma, but the IOL group had significantly more intraoperative and post-operative adverse events and additional intraocular surgeries [25]. Another disadvantage of primary IOL implantation is that the power of the IOL cannot be modified as the eye grows, resulting in potentially large myopic shifts as the child becomes older. In addition, limited by the size of commercially available IOLs, primary implantation may not be possible in very small eyes.

However, as discussed below and also in earlier chapters it is recommended to perform primary IOL implantation in infants older than 6 months with adequate globe size and absence of comorbid ocular conditions.

6.3.2.3 Secondary IOL Implantation

Secondary IOL implantation is usually performed at around 3–5 years of age for those who were left aphakic after cataract extraction, when the growth of the eye can be predicted and the IOL power chosen with more accuracy [26].

6.3.2.4 Involving the Parents in Decision-Making

It is important to discuss the different refractive options thoroughly with the parents before the operation. The authors usually perform primary IOL implantation in infants and children older than 6 months of age with adequate globe size and cornea diameter of at least 9 mm. However, parental concerns, motivation and the likelihood of compliance to refractive and amblyopia treatment should be included in decisions about post-operative refraction in order to optimize visual outcomes. Primary IOL implantation may be considered in infants younger than 6 months of age if compliance to contact lens wear is likely to be unsatisfactory.

6.3.2.5 Refractive Surprise and Myopic Shift

Due to the difficulty of performing accurate biometry and the reduced accuracy of IOL power calculation formulae in children, there is a higher risk of refractive surprise with primary IOL when compared with adults [27]. IOL calculation formulae derived from adult studies fail to take into account the shorter axial length, steeper corneas and shallower anterior chamber depths of children. Moreover, children undergo varying degrees of myopic shift as they grow, resulting in unpredictable refractive errors that require correction.

Myopic Shift

Refractive change in a normal growing eye involves a complex interaction between elongation of axial length, flattening of corneal curvature and reduction in crystalline lens power, resulting in rapid myopic shifts in the first few years of life [28]. Any additional effects on ocular growth by the presence of a congenital cataract, its laterality, age at surgery, post-operative visual input and compliance with post-operative amblyopia therapy remain uncertain. Studies have found large and unpredictable variations in long-term myopic shift following IOL implantation in children, especially when surgery is performed in the first few years of life. At 3-year follow-up after cataract extraction and IOL implantation in infants under the age of 1, refractive change ranged from +2 to −15.5 D in a study by Gouws et al. [29], and from −0.47 to −10.69 D in a study by Fan et al. [30] Larger myopic shifts are associated with younger age at the time of surgery [31–33]. Some studies have also found larger myopic shifts in unilateral cataracts when compared with bilateral cataracts [34, 35].

Optimal Target Refraction for Primary IOL Implantation

Surgeons often aim for initial hyperopia titrated based on age at operation to compensate for the expected myopic shift. This has also been discussed in Chaps. 3 and 4. Table 6.4 shows the suggested target refractions for age by a panel of experts [36]. However, high initial post-operative hyperopia requires good compliance with refractive correction and amblyopia treatment. Hyperopia is particularly amblyogenic, as the child is defocused at both distance and near, especially in pseudophakes due to loss of accommodation. The threat is greater in unilateral cases. Some retrospective studies have found better long-term visual acuity in children with lower (compared with higher) initial post-operative hyperopia [37, 38]. Conversely, aiming for initial post-operative emmetropia will aid amblyopia treatment in the beginning but the eye may eventually become highly myopic. No consensus exists at present, as the magnitude of myopic shift in individual patients remains difficult to predict.

However, lesser under correction of emmetropic IOL power (lesser target hypermetropia) is done in unilateral cataracts, older children and in those with anticipated poor compliance to amblyopia treatment.

Management

Most children will need further refractive correction by spectacles after primary IOL implantation. Some may need contact lenses for high myopia or significant anisometropia. IOL exchange may be considered when there is significant refractive error and poor compliance to refractive correction [39], for example in children with concurrent neurodevelopmental disorders. Others may benefit from corneal refractive surgery when the refractive error becomes stable in adulthood, provided there is sufficient residual corneal thickness. The use of corneal refractive surgery in children remains controversial but may be an option in those who have failed traditional therapies [40]. Piggyback IOLs are also reported to successfully correct the residual refractive error [41].

Several technological innovations have been proposed to address the problem of myopic shift in pediatric pseudophakes. Wilson et al. suggested placing a permanent IOL in the capsular bag and a second "piggy-back" IOL in the ciliary sulcus, which is then removed when myopic shift occurs [42]. However, a retrospective

Table 6.4 Age at cataract surgery and suggested target refraction [32]

Age	Refraction (dioptres)
<6 months	+6 to +10
6–12 months	+4 to +6
1–3 years	+4
3–4 years	+3
4–6 years	+2 to +3
6–8 years	+1 to +2
>8 years	+1 to 0

comparative study found that when compared with primary single IOL implantation in congenital cataract, temporary piggyback IOL implantation produced worse visual acuity, higher re-operation rate and higher risk of secondary glaucoma [43]. Another retrospective study comparing temporary piggyback IOL with aphakia found no difference in visual outcomes but higher rate of re-operation due to complications in the piggyback IOL group [44]. Various types of adjustable IOLs are in development, including those that require secondary surgical procedures (e.g. the multicomponent IOL, the mechanically adjustable IOL and the repeatedly adjustable IOL) and those that can be adjusted non-invasively (e.g. the light-adjustable IOL, the magnetically adjustable IOL, the liquid crystal IOL with wireless control, and IOLs that can be adjusted using femtosecond laser or 2-photon chemistry) [45]. However, these technologies have not been tested in the pediatric population.

6.3.2.6 Loss of Accommodation

Removal of the crystalline lens results in loss of accommodation in children. In infants and younger children, contact lens or spectacles are usually overcorrected by 2.5–3D for best corrected near vision. Older children are corrected for distance and as they enter schooling, varifocal or bifocal glasses are needed.

6.3.3 Corneal Complications

6.3.3.1 Surgically Induced Astigmatism

In pediatric cataract surgery, wounds are typically secured with tight sutures and this can result in large amounts of surgically induced astigmatism in the immediate post-operative period. Associated corneal injuries as seen in traumatic cataracts can further worsen the amount of astigmatism. However, in infants and children, the amount of astigmatism reduces rapidly in the first month as wounds heal and absorbable sutures dissolve [46–48]. Lesser astigmatism is observed in children operated before 3 years of age [48]. Earlier larger wounds were required for insertion of rigid PMMA lenses and scleral tunnels were usually used to reduce the amount of surgically induced astigmatism. Foldable lenses allow the use of smaller main wounds and many surgeons perform clear corneal incisions. When non-absorbable sutures are used and there is significant post-operative astigmatism, timely and selective suture removal is required. Post-operative astigmatism should be carefully monitored and corrected as it can lead to meridional amblyopia in children. Astigmatism can be measured by keratometry or corneal topography in older children but in non-cooperative children retinoscopy can be used to estimate corneal astigmatism, provided there is no significant contribution to astigmatism from IOL tilting or decentration. In most cases, the amount of surgically induced astigmatism is low in the long run and spectacle correction is usually sufficient.

6.3.3.2 Corneal Endothelial Cell Loss and Decompensation

Endothelial cell loss after pediatric cataract surgery has been reported by some authors. At 24–36 weeks after surgery, Basti et al. reported 5.28–7.50% loss of endothelial cells after extracapsular cataract extraction with or without primary posterior capsulotomy and anterior vitrectomy respectively, with no statistically significant difference between the two groups [49]. Using modern surgical techniques and bimanual irrigation and aspiration, Vasavada et al. found a 5.1% decrease in endothelial cell density at 3 months after surgery [50]. However, endothelial cell loss occurs with increasing age even in infants and children. No significant difference in endothelial cell count was found by Nilforushan et al. when operated eyes were compared with age and sex-matched controls [51]. The Infant Aphakia Treatment Study, which studied unilateral congenital cataract in infants, also did not find reduced endothelial cell densities in treated compared to fellow eyes [52]. In both studies, central corneal thickness was increased in the treated eyes. Thicker central corneal thickness is associated with overestimation of intraocular pressure measurements and this should be kept in mind when monitoring for glaucoma.

Corneal decompensation after pediatric cataract surgery is uncommon but the risk is higher for post-traumatic cataracts and cataracts associated with other anterior segment abnormalities or glaucoma. Pre-operative specular microscopy is not routinely performed but may be useful in certain situations, such as secondary intraocular lens implantation, or with associated aniridia and other anterior segment abnormalities. Careful instrumentation and judicious use of ocular viscoelastic devices can reduce intraoperative and subsequent late endothelial cell loss in such situations.

6.3.4 Retinal Detachment

Retinal detachment is a rare complication that can occur any time after pediatric cataract surgery, often many years later (Fig. 6.10). The literature is limited and some of the reports pertain to older surgical techniques for cataract extraction. The mean time interval between cataract surgery and retinal detachment ranged from 6.8 to 33.3 years in different reports [53, 54]. The incidence of retinal detachment was reported to be 3.2% in a series of 1017 eyes of 579 patients with cataract extraction without IOL implantation at the age of 5–16 years, after a mean follow-up of 6.8 years (range 2–18.3 years) [54].

Risk factors for retinal detachment included more myopic aphakic refraction and wound dehiscence. Posterior capsulotomy and anterior vitrectomy were not found to be risk factors. A population-based study of 1043 eyes found an overall 20-year risk of 7%, but only 3% among patients with isolated cataract [55]. A significantly higher risk of retinal detachment was found in children with mental retardation (23%) or in cataracts associated with other ocular or systemic anomalies (16%). A more recent report included surgeries performed between 1996 and 2007 in 481 eyes with no other ocular or systemic anomalies. It found a 5.5% risk for retinal detachment in the first 10 years after cataract surgery [56].

Patients with retinal detachment may present with floaters, flashes, visual field defect or loss of central vision. Presentation may be delayed in young children or in those with pre-existing poor vision. Careful retinal examination should be performed

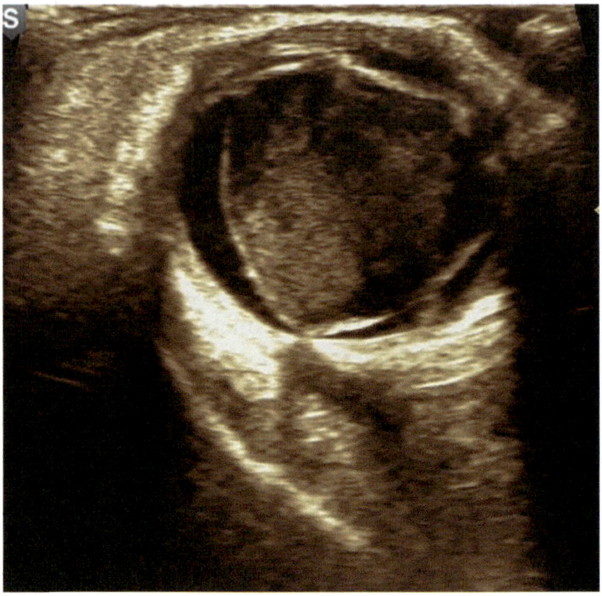

Fig. 6.10 B scan showing retinal detachment (detached 'V' shaped retina attached to optic nerve head) (B Scan image courtesy: Dr. Neha Agarwal, Lucknow, India)

regularly and long-term follow-up is warranted, especially in those with additional risk factors. However, retinal examination can be challenging due to small pupils and peripheral capsular opacities. Early recognition and prompt management are required. Multiple surgeries are needed in a significant proportion of cases [57].

6.3.5 Glaucoma

Glaucoma is a well-recognized complication after congenital cataract surgery. One retrospective study of 170 eyes found that 37.1% of aphakic glaucoma developed by the age of 1 year, but glaucoma can also develop years later, and the prevalence of glaucoma rises with longer duration of follow-up [58]. Onset is bimodal with close-angle glaucoma more common in early-onset cases and open-angle glaucoma in late-onset cases [14, 15]. An increased risk is associated with younger age at surgery, particularly if surgery is performed within the first 4 weeks of life [59, 60]. One retrospective study reported a 5-year risk of glaucoma of 31.6% in eyes operated in the first month of life, compared with 9.3% in eyes operated after the first month of life [58]. Other potential risk factors that have been reported include microcornea, microphthalmia, persistent fetal vasculature, associated ocular anomalies, retained lens material, poor pupil dilatation and history of secondary surgery [56]. The pathogenesis of glaucoma after pediatric cataract surgery is multifactorial. Postulated mechanisms include chronic trabeculitis from inflammation, blockage of the trabecular meshwork by retained lens material, changes in trabecular meshwork due to exposure to lens epithelial cells, exposure to chemical factors from the vitreous, abnormal meshwork development due to loss of normal structural interaction between the native lens, zonules, ciliary body and trabecular meshwork and abnormal anterior segment leading to both cataract and angle anomaly [56].

6.3.5.1 Is Insertion of an IOL Protective?

Some studies suggest that the risk of glaucoma is increased in eyes that are left aphakic after surgery, compared with pseudophakic eyes [61, 62]. However, retrospective studies may be biased by the fact that surgeons tend to implant IOL in older children and more 'normal' eyes, which may lower the observed incidence of glaucoma. Variable durations of follow-up can also confound the results. The randomized controlled trial Infant Aphakic Treatment Study found no difference between the risks of secondary glaucoma in aphakic versus pseudophakic eyes.

6.3.5.2 Monitoring and Diagnosis

As glaucoma can occur any time after surgery, long-term follow-up and regular measurement of intraocular pressure are important. However, since central corneal thickness may increase after cataract surgery, intraocular pressures may be overestimated and the diagnosis of glaucoma cannot be based on intraocular pressure alone. Measurement of central corneal thickness by pachymetry can provide additional information. Assessment for glaucoma in young children is often difficult due to limited cooperation. Children below the age of 3 years may develop buphthalmos. Other signs include corneal clouding, rapid increase in axial length or myopia, optic disc cupping and visual field loss.

6.3.5.3 Treatment

In some children, intraocular pressure may be controlled with medical therapy alone. Options include topical beta-blockers, prostaglandin analogues, carbonic anhydrase inhibitors and alpha 2 agonists. Alpha 2 agonists should be avoided in young children due to risk of central nervous systemic depression, apnoea, bradycardia and hypotension. Beta-blockers are contraindicated in children with asthma or cardiac disease due to risk of bronchospasm and bradycardia. Systemic carbonic anhydrase inhibitors may be required for temporary control of intraocular pressure. Long-term use should be avoided due to systemic side effects. If medical therapy fails, surgical intervention is required. Angle surgery (goniotomy and trabeculotomy) and trabeculectomy with antimetabolites may be effective for some but the success rate is generally poor [63, 64]. Better long-term outcomes have been reported with implantation of glaucoma drainage devices such as Baerveldt and Ahmed valves [65, 66]. Laser cyclophotocoagulation is another option but the effects are temporary. It can be useful for control of intraocular pressure in very young children to buy time before insertion of a glaucoma drainage device. Long-term visual outcomes for aphakic glaucoma can be good although multiple procedures may be needed and some children may continue to require medications after surgery. Bhola et al. found that after a mean follow-up of 18.7 years, 54.5% of children with aphakic glaucoma had a visual acuity of 20/40 or better [67]. A major cause of vision loss in patients with controlled glaucoma is amblyopia.

6.4 Summary

- Cataract surgery carries a higher risk of complications in infants and children than in adults.
- Early post-operative complications include severe inflammation, endophthalmitis, intraocular pressure spike, wound and IOL-related issues. Late complications include visual axis opacification, refractive error, glaucoma, issues-related to cornea and retinal detachment.
- As there is a lifelong risk of developing complications, children need to be followed long-term.
- It is essential to inform parents about these risks and make them understand the importance of post-operative care and follow-up.
- Early diagnosis and proper management of complications are important to ensure good long-term outcomes.

Multiple Choice Questions

1. Which of the following is associated with the lowest incidence of posterior capsular opacification in infants?
   (a) Primary posterior capsulotomy and anterior vitrectomy
   (b) Primary posterior capsulotomy, no anterior vitrectomy
   (c) Primary anterior vitrectomy only, no posterior capsulotomy
   (d) No posterior capsulotomy or anterior vitrectomy

   Answer: *(a) Primary posterior capsulotomy and anterior vitrectomy.* Lens epithelial cells may migrate and proliferate on the anterior vitreous surface causing visual axis opacification. Hence primary posterior capsulotomy should be combined with anterior vitrectomy in infants.

2. Which of the following clinical signs is present in endophthalmitis but NOT in toxic anterior segment syndrome (TASS)?
   (a) Corneal oedema
   (b) Fibrin formation
   (c) Hypopyon
   (d) Vitritis

   Answer: *(d) Vitritis.* Vitritis is a differentiating feature between the two conditions. If view of the posterior segment is not possible, B scan ultrasound should be used to evaluate inflammation in the vitreous humour.

3. Which of the following risk factors is most strongly associated with the development of glaucoma after pediatric cataract surgery?
   (a) Aphakia
   (b) Surgery performed within the first 4 weeks of life
   (c) Persistent fetal vasculature
   (d) Poor pupil dilatation

Answer: *(b) Surgery performed within the first 4 weeks of life.* While other conditions are also associated with glaucoma, surgery within the first 4 weeks has the strongest association.

4. Which of the following can lead to elevated intraocular pressure measurements after pediatric cataract surgery?
   (a) Glaucoma
   (b) Thick central corneal thickness
   (c) Steroid response
   (d) All of the above

   Answer: *(d) All of the above.* While glaucoma and steroid response cause raised intraocular pressure, thickened cornea leads to falsely high readings.

5. What of the following is NOT a risk factor for retinal detachment following pediatric cataract surgery?
   (a) Wound dehiscence
   (b) Posterior capsulotomy and anterior vitrectomy
   (c) Mental retardation
   (d) Cataracts associated with other ocular or systemic anomalies

   Answer: *(b) Posterior capsulotomy and anterior vitrectomy.* While all other conditions are associated with increased occurrence of retinal detachment, posterior capsulotomy and anterior vitrectomy are not.

References

1. Nihalani BR, Vanderveen DK. Secondary intraocular lens implantation after pediatric aphakia. J Am Assoc Pediatr Ophthalmol Strabismus. 2011;15(5):435–40. https://doi.org/10.1016/j.jaapos.2011.05.019.
2. Phatak S, Lowder C, Pavesio C. Controversies in intraocular lens implantation in pediatric uveitis. J Ophthalmic Inflamm Infect. 2016;6(1):12. https://doi.org/10.1186/s12348-016-0079-y.
3. Wilson ME, Elliott L, Johnson B, et al. AcrySof acrylic intraocular lens implantation in children: clinical indications of biocompatibility. J Am Assoc Pediatr Ophthalmol Strabismus. 2001;5(6):377–80. https://doi.org/10.1067/mpa.2001.119786.
4. Bayramlar H, Totan Y, Borazan M. Heparin in the intraocular irrigating solution in pediatric cataract surgery. J Cataract Refract Surg. 2004;30(10):2163–9.
5. Mehta JS, Adams GG. Recombinant tissue plasminogen activator following paediatric cataract surgery. Br J Ophthalmol. 2000;84(9):983–6.
6. Klais CM, Hattenbach LO, Steinkamp GW, Zubcov AA, Kohnen T. Intraocular recombinant tissue-plasminogen activator fibrinolysis of fibrin formation after cataract surgery in children. J Cataract Refract Surg. 1999;25(3):357–62.
7. Huang Y, Dai Y, Wu X, Lan J, Xie L. Toxic anterior segment syndrome after pediatric cataract surgery. J Am Assoc Pediatr Ophthalmol Strabismus. 2010;14(5):444–6.
8. Ari Ş, Caca İ, Sahin A, Cingü AK. Toxic anterior segment syndrome subsequent to pediatric cataract surgery. Cutan Ocul Toxicol. 2012;31(1):53–7.

9. Wheeler DT, Stager DR, Weakley DR. Endophthalmitis following pediatric intraocular surgery for congenital cataracts and congenital glaucoma. J Pediatr Ophthalmol Strabismus. 1992;29(3):139–41.
10. Good WV, Hing S, Irvine AR, Hoyt CS, Taylor DS. Postoperative endophthalmitis in children following cataract surgery. J Pediatr Ophthalmol Strabismus. 1990;27(6):283–5.
11. Al-Rashaed SA, Abu El-Asrar AM. Exogenous endophthalmitis in pediatric age group. Ocul Immunol Inflamm. 2006;14(5):285–92.
12. Zhang M, Xu G-Z, Jiang R, et al. Pediatric infectious endophthalmitis: a 271-case retrospective study at a single center in China. Chin Med J. 2016;129(24):2936–43.
13. Dave H, Phoenix V, Becker ER, Lambert SR. Simultaneous vs sequential bilateral cataract surgery for infants with congenital cataracts: visual outcomes, adverse events, and economic costs. Arch Ophthalmol. 2010;128(8):1050–4.
14. Agrawal S, Singh V, Vinod Kumar BM, Meena M, Srivastava RM, Katiyar V. Immediate sequential bilateral cataract surgery in children in a government medical university in India. J Clin Ophthalmol Res. 2020;8:14–7.
15. Tehrani M, Dick HB, Krummenauer F, Pfirrman G, Boyle T, Stoffelns BM. Capsule measuring ring to predict capsular bag diameter and follow its course after foldable intraocular lens implantation. J Cataract Refract Surg. 2003;29(11):2127–34.
16. Kumar DA, Agarwal A, Prakash D, Prakash G, Jacob S, Agarwal A. Glued Intrascleral Fixation of posterior chamber intraocular lens in children. Am J Ophthalmol. 2012;153(4):594–601.e2.
17. Kang KD, Bin Yim H, Biglan AW. Comparison of delayed-onset glaucoma and early-onset glaucoma after infantile cataract surgery. Korean J Ophthalmol. 2006;20(1):41–6.
18. Mills MD, Robb RM. Glaucoma following childhood cataract surgery, J Pediatr Ophthalmol Strabismus. 1994;31(6):355–60; discussion 361
19. Vasavada AR, Praveen MR, Tassignon M-J, et al. Posterior capsule management in congenital cataract surgery. J Cataract Refract Surg. 2011;37(1):173–93.
20. Hutcheson KA, Drack AV, Ellish NJ, Lambert SR. Anterior hyaloid face opacification after pediatric Nd:YAG laser capsulotomy. J Am Assoc Pediatr Ophthalmol Strabismus. 1999;3(5):303–7. https://doi.org/10.1016/S1091-8531(99)70027-3.
21. Ahmadieh H, Javadi MA, Ahmady M, et al. Primary capsulectomy, anterior vitrectomy, lensectomy, and posterior chamber lens implantation in children: limbal versus pars plana. J Cataract Refract Surg. 1999;25(6):768–75.
22. Tassignon MJ, De Veuster I, Godts D, Kosec D, Van den Dooren K, Gobin L. Bag-in-the-lens intraocular lens implantation in the pediatric eye. J Cataract Refract Surg. 2007;33(4):611–7.
23. Jensen AA, Basti S, Greenwald MJ, Mets MB. When may the posterior capsule be preserved in pediatric intraocular lens surgery? Ophthalmology. 2002;109(2):324–7. discussion 328
24. Whitman MC, Vanderveen DK. Complications of pediatric cataract surgery. Semin Ophthalmol. 2014;29(5-6):414–20.
25. Lambert SR, Lynn MJ, Hartmann EE, et al. Comparison of contact lens and intraocular lens correction of monocular aphakia during infancy. JAMA Ophthalmol. 2014;132(6):676.
26. Wood KS, Tadros D, Trivedi RH, Wilson ME. Secondary intraocular lens implantation following infantile cataract surgery: intraoperative indications, postoperative outcomes. Eye. 2016;30(9):1182–6.
27. O'Hara MA. Pediatric intraocular lens power calculations. Curr Opin Ophthalmol. 2012;23(5):388–93.
28. Gordon RA, Donzis PB. Refractive development of the human eye. Arch Ophthalmol (Chicago, Ill 1960). 1985;103(6):785–9.
29. Gouws P, Hussin HM, Markham RHC. Long term results of primary posterior chamber intraocular lens implantation for congenital cataract in the first year of life. Br J Ophthalmol. 2006;90(8):975–8.
30. Fan DSP, Rao SK, Yu CBO, Wong CY, Lam DSC. Changes in refraction and ocular dimensions after cataract surgery and primary intraocular lens implantation in infants. J Cataract Refract Surg. 2006;32(7):1104–8.

31. Crouch ER, Crouch ER, Pressman SH. Prospective analysis of pediatric pseudophakia: myopic shift and postoperative outcomes. J AAPOS Off Publ Am Assoc Pediatr Ophthalmol Strabismus. 2002;6(5):277–82.
32. Hoevenaars NED, Polling JR, Wolfs RCW. Prediction error and myopic shift after intraocular lens implantation in paediatric cataract patients. Br J Ophthalmol. 2011;95(8):1082–5.
33. Dahan E, Drusedau MU. Choice of lens and dioptric power in pediatric pseudophakia. J Cataract Refract Surg. 1997;23(Suppl 1):618–23.
34. Negalur M, Sachdeva V, Neriyanuri S, Ali M, Kekunnaya R. Long-term outcomes following primary intraocular lens implantation in infants younger than 6 months. Indian J Ophthalmol. 2018;66(8):1088.
35. McClatchey SK, Dahan E, Maselli E, et al. A comparison of the rate of refractive growth in pediatric aphakic and pseudophakic eyes. Ophthalmology. 2000;107(1):118–22.
36. Serafino M, Trivedi RH, Levin AV, et al. Use of the Delphi process in paediatric cataract management. Br J Ophthalmol. 2016;100(5):611–5.
37. Magli A, Forte R, Carelli R, Rombetto L, Magli G. Long-term outcomes of primary intraocular lens implantation for unilateral congenital cataract. Semin Ophthalmol. 2015;31(6):1–6.
38. Lowery RS, Nick TG, Shelton JB, Warner D, Green T. Long-term visual acuity and initial postoperative refractive error in pediatric pseudophakia. Can J Ophthalmol. 2011;46(2):143–7.
39. Kraus CL, Trivedi RH, Wilson ME. Intraocular lens exchange for high myopia in pseudophakic children. Eye. 2016;30(9):1199–203.
40. Stahl ED. Pediatric refractive surgery. Pediatr Clin N Am. 2014;61(3):519–27.
41. Agrawal S, Singh V, Yadav A, Katiyar V. Orthoptic relevance of refractive correction in the phakic plane in unilateral high refractive errors in adults. Oman J Ophthalmol. 2016;9:196–8.
42. Wilson ME, Peterseim MW, Englert JA, Lall-Trail JK, Elliott LA. Pseudophakia and polypseudophakia in the first year of life. J Am Assoc Pediatr Ophthalmol Strabismus. 2001;5(4):238–45.
43. Hwang S, Lim DH, Lee S, Choi DD, Chung E-S, Chung T-Y. Temporary piggyback intraocular lens implantation versus single intraocular lens implantation in congenital cataracts: long-term clinical outcomes. Investig Opthalmology Vis Sci. 2018;59(5):1822.
44. Joshaghani M, Soleimani M, Foroutan A, Yaseri M. Visual outcomes and complications of piggyback intraocular lens implantation compared to aphakia for infantile cataract. Middle East Afr J Ophthalmol. 2015;22(4):495.
45. Ford J, Werner L, Mamalis N. Adjustable intraocular lens power technology. J Cataract Refract Surg. 2014;40(7):1205–23.
46. Spierer A, Nahum A. Changes in astigmatism after congenital cataract surgery and intraocular lens implantation using scleral tunnel incision. Eye. 2002;16(4):466–8.
47. Bothun ED, Johnson CS, Archer SM, Del Monte MA. Evolution of postoperative astigmatism after large incision PMMA lens implantation in children. J AAPOS Off Publ Am Assoc Pediatr Ophthalmol Strabismus. 2010;14(6):518–21.
48. Bradfield YS, Plager DA, Neely DE, Sprunger DT, Sondhi N. Astigmatism after small-incision clear corneal cataract extraction and intraocular lens implantation in children. J Cataract Refract Surg. 2004;30(9):1948–52.
49. Basti S, Aasuri MK, Reddy S, Reddy S, Rao GN. Prospective evaluation of corneal endothelial cell loss after pediatric cataract surgery. J Cataract Refract Surg. 1998;24(11):1469–73.
50. Vasavada AR, Praveen MR, Vasavada VA, Shah SK, Vasavada V, Trivedi RH. Corneal endothelial morphologic assessment in pediatric cataract surgery with intraocular lens implantation: a comparison of preoperative and early postoperative specular microscopy. Am J Ophthalmol. 2012;154(2):259–265.e1.
51. Nilforushan N, Falavarjani KG, Razeghinejad MR, Bakhtiari P. Cataract surgery for congenital cataract: endothelial cell characteristics, corneal thickness, and impact on intraocular pressure. J AAPOS Off Publ Am Assoc Pediatr Ophthalmol Strabismus. 2007;11(2):159–61.

52. Morrison DG, Lynn MJ, Freedman SF, Orge FH, Lambert SR. Infant Aphakia Treatment Study Group. Corneal changes in children after unilateral cataract surgery in the Infant Aphakia Treatment Study. Ophthalmology. 2015;122(11):2186–92.
53. Rabiah PK, Du H, Hahn EA. Frequency and predictors of retinal detachment after pediatric cataract surgery without primary intraocular lens implantation. J AAPOS Off Publ Am Assoc Pediatr Ophthalmol Strabismus. 2005;9(2):152–9.
54. Kanski JJ, Elkington AR, Daniel R. Retinal detachment after congenital cataract surgery. Br J Ophthalmol. 1974;58(2):92–5.
55. Haargaard B, Andersen EW, Oudin A, et al. Risk of retinal detachment after pediatric cataract surgery. Investig Opthalmology Vis Sci. 2014;55(5):2947.
56. Agarkar S, Gokhale VV, Raman R, Bhende M, Swaminathan G, Jain M. Incidence, risk factors, and outcomes of retinal detachment after pediatric cataract surgery. Ophthalmology. 2018;125(1):36–42.
57. Yorston D, Yang YF, Sullivan PM. Retinal detachment following surgery for congenital cataract: presentation and outcomes. Eye (Lond). 2005;19(3):317–21.
58. Chen TC, Walton DS, Bhatia LS. Aphakic glaucoma after congenital cataract surgery. Arch Ophthalmol. 2004;122(12):1819.
59. Watts P, Abdolell M, Levin AV. Complications in infants undergoing surgery for congenital cataract in the first 12 weeks of life: is early surgery better? J AAPOS Off Publ Am Assoc Pediatr Ophthalmol Strabismus. 2003;7(2):81–5.
60. Vishwanath M, Cheong-Leen R, Taylor D, Russell-Eggitt I, Rahi J. Is early surgery for congenital cataract a risk factor for glaucoma? Br J Ophthalmol. 2004;88(7):905–10.
61. Asrani S, Freedman S, Hasselblad V, et al. Does primary intraocular lens implantation prevent "aphakic" glaucoma in children? J AAPOS Off Publ Am Assoc Pediatr Ophthalmol Strabismus. 2000;4(1):33–9.
62. Zhang S, Wang J, Li Y, Liu Y, He L, Xia X. The role of primary intraocular lens implantation in the risk of secondary glaucoma following congenital cataract surgery: A systematic review and meta-analysis. PLoS One. 2019;14(4):e0214684.
63. Bothun ED, Guo Y, Christiansen SP, et al. Outcome of angle surgery in children with aphakic glaucoma. J Am Assoc Pediatr Ophthalmol Strabismus. 2010;14(3):235–9.
64. Mandal AK, Bagga H, Nutheti R, Gothwal VK, Nanda AK. Trabeculectomy with or without mitomycin-C for paediatric glaucoma in aphakia and pseudophakia following congenital cataract surgery. Eye. 2003;17(1):53–62.
65. Kirwan C, O'Keefe M, Lanigan B, Mahmood U. Ahmed valve drainage implant surgery in the management of paediatric aphakic glaucoma. Br J Ophthalmol. 2005;89(7):855–8.
66. van Overdam KA, de Faber JTHN, Lemij HG, de Waard PWT. Baerveldt glaucoma implant in paediatric patients. Br J Ophthalmol. 2006;90(3):328–32.
67. Bhola R, Keech RV, Olson RJ, Petersen DB. Long-Term Outcome of Pediatric Aphakic Glaucoma. J Am Assoc Pediatr Ophthalmol Strabismus. 2006;10(3):243–8.

Considerations in Traumatic Cataract in Children

7

Ramesh Kekunnaya and Rajat Kapoor

7.1 Introduction

Ocular injuries have a wide spectrum of presentations ranging from trivial corneal abrasion to vision-threatening retinal detachment. Many a time, injuries are preventable and such occurrences in children can lead to life-long handicaps with huge socioeconomic burden on the society. Traumatic cataracts account for 29% of all childhood cataracts [1]. Traumatic cataracts are commonly associated with other ocular injuries like corneo-scleral tears, iris injury, lens subluxation or dislocation, vitreous haemorrhage, and retinal tears [2]. Managing traumatic cataracts in children is a daunting task requiring highest levels of clinical skills and cooperation between various ophthalmological subspecialties.

This chapter will cover the classification of ocular trauma, mechanism of involvement of crystalline lens, clinical evaluation of a child with ocular trauma and considerations for decision-making. Relevant surgical steps, complications and follow-up protocol would also be discussed.

7.2 Epidemiology and Significance of Traumatic Cataract in Children

A large proportion (20–50%) of all ocular injuries occur in children. In India, one of the most common causes of childhood blindness is cataract [3]. Traumatic cataract is common in children with an average age of about 6 years [4]. It is commoner in boys because they often engage in sports, play without wearing protective gear and

R. Kekunnaya (✉) · R. Kapoor
Child Sight Institute, LV Prasad Eye Institute, Hyderabad, India
e-mail: rameshak@lvpei.org

S. Agrawal (ed.), *Pediatric Cataract*,
https://doi.org/10.1007/978-981-16-1736-2_7

without supervision. Penetrating injuries account for about 75% of cases [4]. The commonly involved objects associated with ocular injury in children are wooden sticks, pencils, sharp metallic objects, scissors, stones, balls, firecrackers, toys, bow and arrow etc. [5].

The management of these cases is challenging because of the associated ocular comorbidities. Also, multiple surgeries may be needed which are often time consuming and expensive. Despite modern surgical techniques, instruments and better methods of lens power calculation problems related to changes in axial length, developing visual structures, need of general anaesthesia for every procedure and risk of amblyopia makes these cases more difficult to manage compared to adults [6–9].

The chief strategy to prevent ocular injury is to gain knowledge about the possible causes of injury and sensitize parents and school staff about the same. Overall, eye trauma represents a very sizable and potentially preventable burden on both victims and society as a whole [10]. Prevention of eye injuries is of paramount importance and any strategy devised regarding this should involve a team of family, teachers, sports coaches, ophthalmologists, pediatricians, radiologists and optometrists.

7.3 Classification of Ocular Trauma

A standardized system has been designed for reporting mechanical injury associated with open- and closed-globe trauma by the ***Ocular Trauma Classification Group***. This system is based on the type of injury, grade (based on visual acuity), zone (based on area involved) and presence or absence of an afferent pupillary defect [11, 12]. The classification predicts the visual outcome after management.

Another system being commonly followed for describing ocular trauma is the ***Birmingham Eye Trauma Terminology System (BETT)***, which is a comprehensive system of eye trauma-related terms and has divided eye trauma into closed and open globe trauma [9]. The BETT has been depicted in Table 7.1.

Table 7.1 BETT classification of ocular trauma

Closed Globe
• Contusion
• Lamellar laceration
Open Globe
• Rupture
• Laceration
Penetration
Perforation
Intraocular foreign body (IOFB)

7.3.1 Closed Globe Trauma

Absence of a full-thickness wound in either cornea or sclera (outer coats) where none of the intraocular contents have been exposed is labelled as a closed-globe injury. Mechanisms of closed globe injury are:

1. **Contusion:** A blunt force may cause ocular injury by following mechanisms:
   (a) Coup mechanism involves local injury via direct impact. The imprint of iris pigments on the anterior lens capsule *(Vossius ring)* following blunt trauma is an example of coup injury (Fig. 7.1).
   (b) Contre-coup mechanism causes distant injury usually at the opposite end of the globe, not by direct contact but due to shock waves traversing along the line of direct contact.
   (c) Equatorial expansion due to anterior-posterior shortening of the eyeball occurs when anterior surface of the eye is compressed with force by a blunt object. The equatorial expansion may cause damage to the zonule-lens complex.
2. **Lamellar laceration:** This is a partial thickness laceration caused by a sharp object.

A closed globe injury could be due to a combination of the above mechanisms and may even be associated with a superficial (extraocular) foreign body.

7.3.2 Open Globe Trauma

An open globe injury is a full-thickness wound exposing the intraocular contents. Open globe injuries can be further subdivided as:

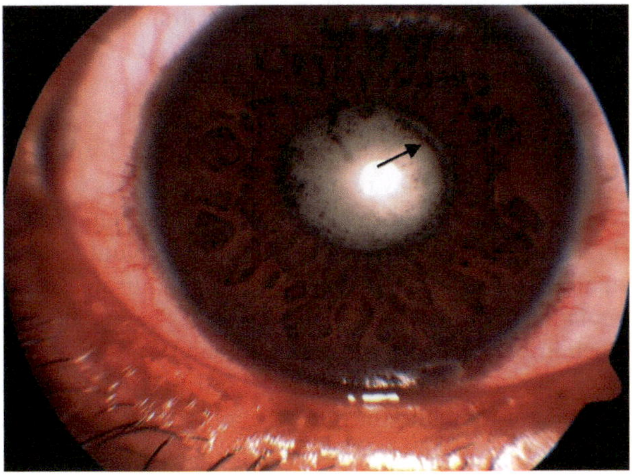

Fig. 7.1 Vossius ring-iris pigment imprint on anterior lens capsule

1. **Rupture:** Globe rupture occurs when a blunt object striking the eyeball results in a full-thickness breach in the outer coats along with expulsion of the contents of the eye. The blow causes a sudden, rapid increase in intraocular pressure (IOP) resulting in rupture of the globe from within out.
2. **Laceration:** Unlike globe rupture, laceration is caused by a sharp object as it breaches the outer coats while entering the eye. The direction of the force is from out to inside of the eye. The margins at the entry site are usually irregular and it may be full thickness at some locations and partial thickness at others. It is further classified into the following subtypes:
   (a) **Penetrating injury:** This includes a single full-thickness laceration of the eye wall usually caused by a sharp object. There is no exit wound in these types of injuries. If more than one entry wounds are present, they are caused by different objects.
   (b) **Intraocular foreign body (IOFB):** Often, penetrating injuries of the eye may be associated with a retained intraocular foreign body. These are often metallic or wooden in nature and usually represent the retained bits of the object causing injury. These injuries are classified separately as presence of IOFB not only compromises the prognosis but also complicates the management of a penetrating injury.
   (c) **Perforating injury:** This type of injury has two full-thickness lacerations with an entry and exit wound caused by the same agent.

7.4 Traumatic Cataract

The crystalline lens is one of the most commonly involved structures in any case of ocular trauma. Traumatic cataract could be an immediate, early, or late sequel of any ocular trauma. Both, closed globe and open globe injuries can cause traumatic cataract. However, the mechanisms, associated injuries and the morphology of cataract may vary depending upon the type of injury.

In closed globe injuries, a combination of coup, countercoup and equatorial expansion of eyeball following blunt trauma is responsible for the formation of traumatic cataract. Furthermore, equatorial expansion of the eye may damage the lens–zonule complex resulting in varying extent of zonular dialysis and lens subluxation. There may be different cataract morphologies associated with blunt trauma. Cataracts post-blunt trauma characteristically form rosette-shaped (Fig. 7.2) opacity of the lens, which may remain stable or progress with time. An anterior lens capsular scar or a fibrosed white anterior lens capsule may be seen at the site of direct impact (Fig. 7.3). Traumatic mydriasis following blunt trauma occurs due to the multiple small ruptures of the pupillary sphincter muscles and may be associated with lenticular opacities (Fig. 7.4). The pupil may be mid dilated, non-reacting or sluggishly reacting and may retain its original round configuration at times. A *Vossius ring* may also be seen associated with cataract following blunt trauma (Fig. 7.1).

Penetrating injury that directly compromises the lens capsule following entry via cornea or sclera often leads to lens opacification at the site of injury (Fig. 7.5). If

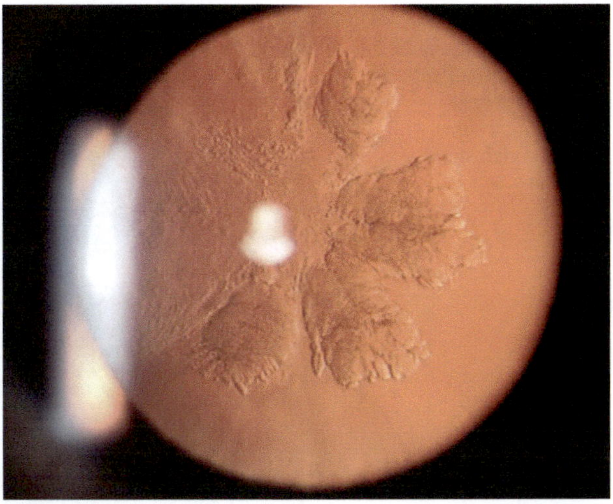

Fig. 7.2 Rosette shaped lenticular opacification post-blunt trauma

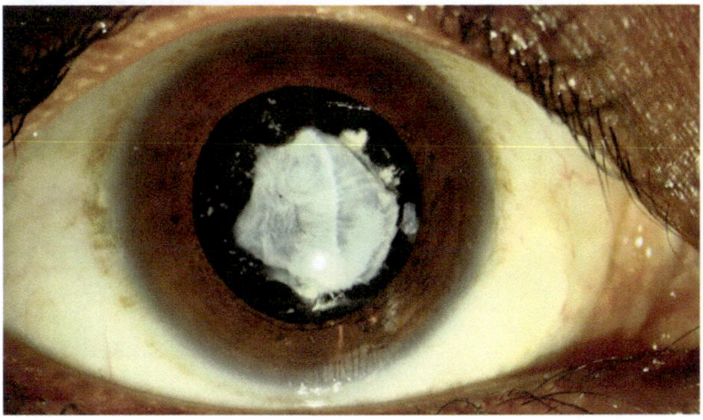

Fig. 7.3 Anterior lens capsular fibrosis

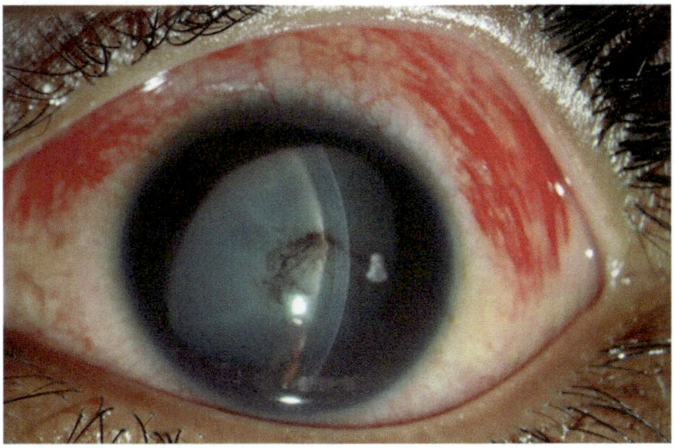

Fig. 7.4 Traumatic mydriasis due to rupture of pupillary sphincter muscles post-blunt trauma

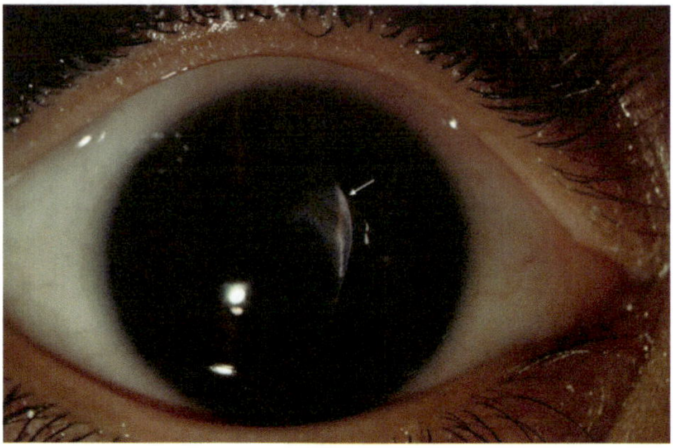

Fig. 7.5 Localized lenticular opacity in the area of rupture of anterior lens capsule post-penetrating trauma with sharp wooden stick fragment

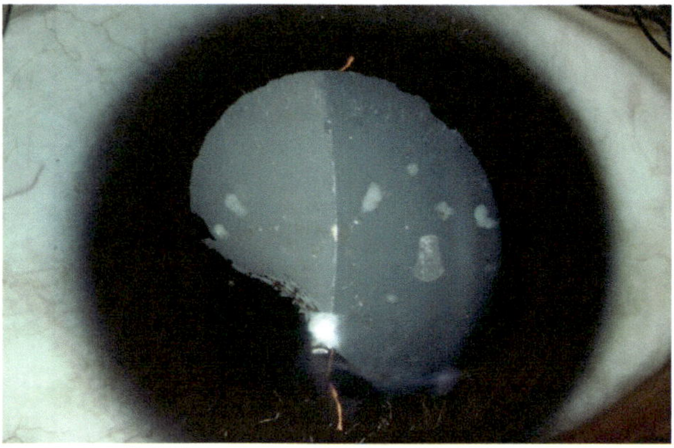

Fig. 7.6 Total lenticular opacification

the capsular entry is sufficiently large, the entire lens rapidly opacifies as it imbibes fluid from the aqueous or vitreous humor (Fig. 7.6). In some cases, when the capsular entry is small, the cataract may remain localized, especially if the entry site is blocked by the agent causing the trauma.

As mentioned earlier with closed globe injury, various components of the crystalline lens–zonule complex may also be affected in penetrating traumas:

- Anterior and/or posterior capsule defect (Fig. 7.7)
- Intra-lenticular foreign body
- Zonular injury (Fig. 7.8)
- Lens dislocation
- Lens subluxation (Fig. 7.9)

Anterior capsule may also be ruptured in open globe injuries with the release of cortical matter from the crystalline lens into the anterior chamber (Fig. 7.10). Other ocular comorbidities associated with traumatic cataract may include:

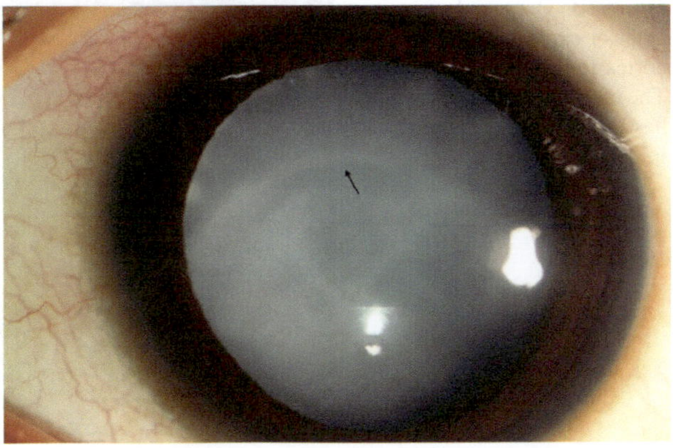

Fig. 7.7 Posterior capsular rupture post trauma (demarcated by the arrow)

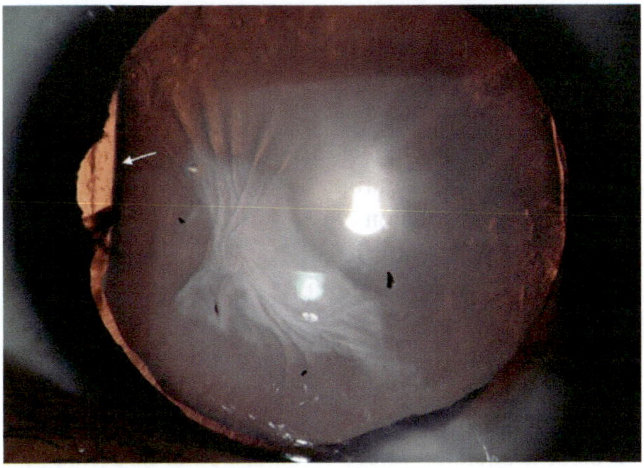

Fig. 7.8 Zonulodialysis seen in 4 clock hours (arrow) along with a cataractous lens

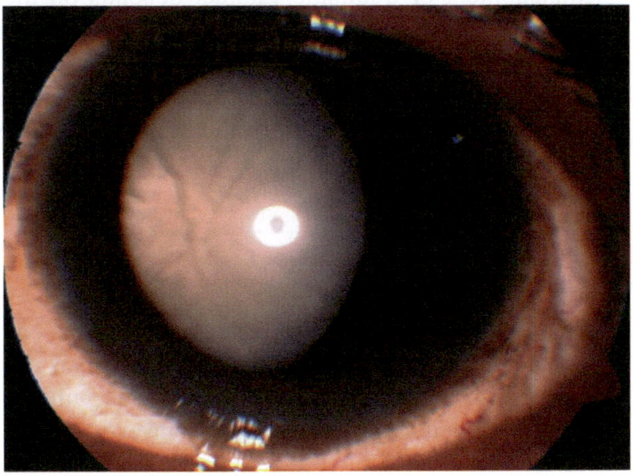

Fig. 7.9 Subluxated cataractous lens

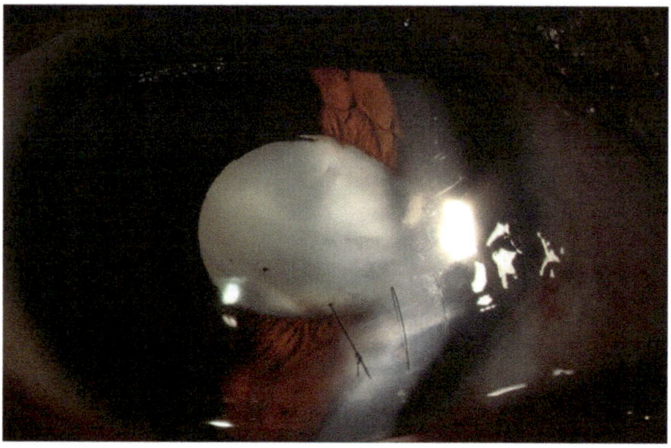

Fig. 7.10 Breached anterior capsule with fluffy cortex in anterior chamber. The entry wound in cornea has been repaired in the initial surgery

- Hyphema and associated corneal staining
- Glaucoma (phacolytic, phacomorphic, pupillary block and angle recession)
- Traumatic iridocyclitis
- Retinal detachment
- Choroidal rupture
- Vitreous haemorrhage
- Traumatic optic neuropathy
- Optic nerve avulsion
- Retrobulbar haemorrhage
- Globe rupture/perforation

Due to high association of associated ocular injuries, a detailed ocular examination including relevant investigations should be performed even if a traumatic cataract is visible in plain sight [13]. The cataract surgeon should always be suspicious of associated injury to other ocular structures and plan accordingly to tackle per-operative untoward incidents.

Management of traumatic cataract depends on the degree and type of injury. Localized traumatic cataracts (especially if not in the visual axis) or small capsular breaches may be managed conservatively, with a close follow-up. Frequently, such injuries develop a much-localized opacification of the underlying cortex which may not be progressive. More significant lens opacities, especially ones that obstruct the visual axis require early surgery.

7.5 Clinical Evaluation

A detailed and comprehensive patient evaluation is one of the most important steps in the management of ocular trauma. This involves recording the exact history followed by initial examination. Information thus gathered helps the treating physician decide the immediate priorities, further investigations, further course of action and the prognosis.

7.5.1 History of Injury

The history should include a description of the circumstances and time of injury. The force and mechanism of injury may give clues about the severity of injury, whether an occult perforation, intraocular foreign body or coexisting posterior segment trauma may exist. For example, an intraocular metallic foreign body is highly probable in chisel and hammer injury. Similarly, injury with vegetative matter is likely to be infectious. It must be remembered that history given by children may often be unreliable. Sometimes, the traumatic cataract presents months or years after the injury when the actual event may have been forgotten. Implications of these for the clinician are to remain suspicious and be prepared for all possibilities.

7.5.2 Examination

A comprehensive ocular examination includes pre- and post-dilatation examinations. Efforts must be made to make the child comfortable and relaxed during the examination. Forcing the examination by overcoming opposition is usually counterproductive and may increase the trauma to the eye.

(a) **Pre-dilatation examination:**

Specific points that should not be missed on a torchlight and slit lamp examination include:

- Best-corrected visual acuity (BCVA): Measuring the uncorrected visual acuity and BCVA may be tedious with the requirement of age appropriate methods (Table 3.4). However, this should never be missed as it affects the management and prognosis. It is also important from medico-legal aspect in patients with trauma.
- Fixation: How readily the injured eye fixes on torchlight is indicative of its vision. This is specifically useful in children who are uncooperative for visual assessment by subjective methods. It has been discussed in Chap. 3 and correlates with Snellen acuity [14].
- Orbital margins should be palpated to rule out any obvious bone injury.
- Ocular malalignment may indicate injury to the extra-ocular muscles or their nerve supply. It may also occur in a long-standing deviation and indicate poor prognosis.
- Extra-ocular motility should be checked to rule out injury to extra-ocular muscles, their nerve supply and orbital soft tissue.
- Pupillary reflex: The presence of an afferent pupillary defect may be indicative of optic nerve injury.
- IOP should be estimated preferably with rebound tonometry, but only in closed globe injuries.
- Siedel test should be performed when there is doubt about the wound integrity.
- Anterior chamber: Irregularity in anterior chamber depth should be specifically looked for which may point towards lens subluxation/dislocation or occult iridodialysis.

- Iris: Trans-illumination defects in iris or tears in the pupillary sphincter with corresponding breach in anterior capsule of lens suggest IOFB or penetrating injury (Figs. 7.11 and 7.12).
- Zonules: Although zonules cannot be visualized pre dilatation, presence of iridodonesis or phacodonesis, increase in myopic astigmatism, abnormal peripheral lens curvature, asymmetrical Bruckner reflex, visible lens equator in the pupillary axis or vitreous in the anterior chamber indicates possible zonular damage. The extent of zonular damage is confirmed after dilatation.

(b) **Post-dilatation Examination**

Examination after dilation should include:

- Detailed slit-lamp examination, if feasible, after appropriately positioning the patient. This helps to identity (and document) the type of cataract, lens

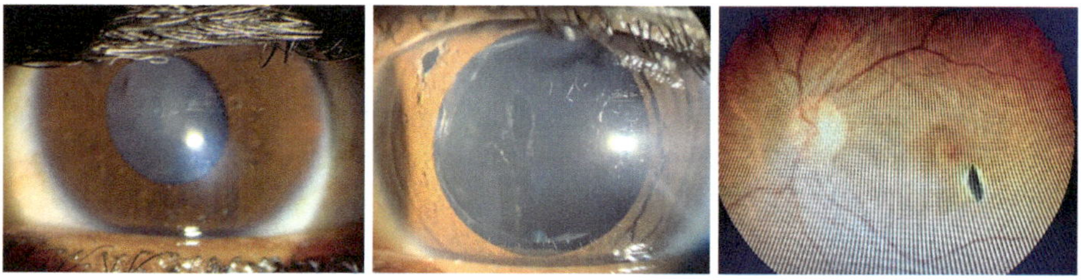

Fig. 7.11 (L to R) Sequelae of chisel and hammer injury with a metallic projectile. Breach in anterior capsule with cataractous changes in crystalline lens. Post-operative image after lens aspiration and implantation of PCIOL showing a defect in iris and an opening in the posterior capsule. The metallic foreign body was lodged in the macular region of the retina (Photograph courtesy: Dr. Mohit Khattri, Kanpur, India)

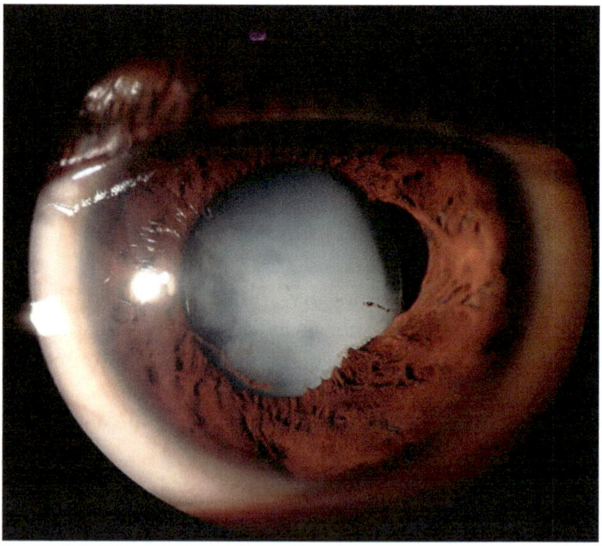

Fig. 7.12 Sphincter tear with subluxation of cataractous lens

capsule integrity, position/stability of the lens, signs like iridodonesis or phacodonesis and any other abnormalities of the anterior segment. In non-ambulatory/uncooperative patients a portable handheld slit lamp in a supine position or an operating microscope may be used after sedation.

- Close attention should be given to the pupillary sphincter muscles, anterior chamber depth and presence of any foreign body in cornea/anterior chamber/angles (gonioscopy)/on the iris or anterior lens surface. Anterior lens surface should also be examined for iris pigments (Vossius ring) in blunt trauma.
- A complete posterior segment examination using indirect ophthalmoscope, including examination of the retinal periphery, should be carried if media clarity allows. In presence of total traumatic cataract or limited view of posterior segment due to any other cause, B-scan ultrasonography should essentially be done before surgery.
- Gonioscopy should be carefully done for evaluating angle structures for possible angle recession, foreign bodies and vitreous prolapse through zonulodialysis. Gonioscopy should be performed both pre and post dilatation. However, it should be avoided in acute trauma.

7.6 Investigations

Appropriate imaging (X Rays and CT Scan) should be carried out when injury to the orbital walls or presence of a foreign body is suspected. B scan ultrasonography is mandatory when a proper view of posterior segment is obscured for any reason (Fig. 7.13). Ultrasound biomicroscopy (UBM) is helpful in the examination of anterior segment in presence of media opacities. It identifies cyclodialysis, subluxation of crystalline lens and presence of a foreign body [15].

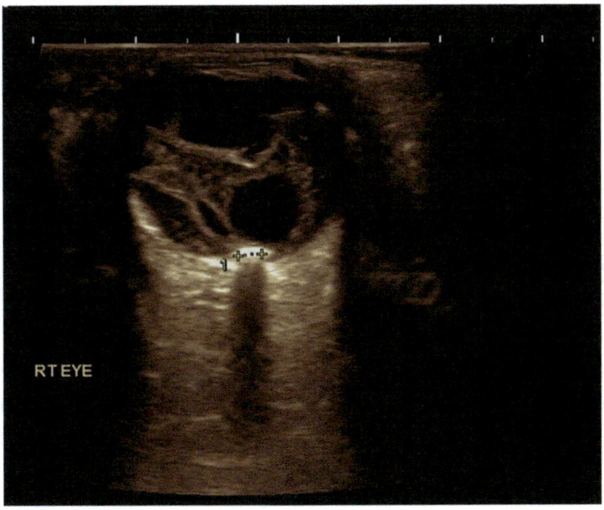

Fig. 7.13 Intraocular foreign body (IOFB) marked by ++ visualized on B Scan (Image courtesy: Dr. Neha Agarwal, Lucknow, India)

When an intraocular lens (IOL) implantation is planned automated keratometry, immersion A-scan ultrasound for axial length and anterior chamber depth measurements are performed. In non-ambulatory patients, a handheld keratometer may be used. Children who are uncooperative, require examination under anaesthesia, which may be planned along with the primary surgery (corneal/scleral repair). Even in presence of corneal irregularity, keratometry of the injured eye should be attempted. Multiple readings should be taken to achieve maximum accuracy. Measurements of the fellow eye may be used as a last resort, keeping in mind the compromised accuracy of post-operative refraction [16]. Changes in corneal curvature due to injury or its repair may affect the refractive outcome often warranting IOL implantation as a secondary procedure. These have also been discussed in earlier chapters.

7.7 Preoperative Counselling

Counselling of the patient and attendants is a critical part of the management of ocular injures. Also, appropriate documentation and recording of medico-legal case (MLC) reports should be done in suspicious cases. A guarded visual prognosis for both anatomical and functional outcomes should be thoroughly explained to the patient (if old enough) and the guardians. Some important points to be explained are:

- Need for photographic and detailed documentation.
- Need for proper consent/MLC forms.
- Need for complete examination which may need sedation or even anaesthesia. The parents should be aware that despite best efforts, the full extent of the ocular injuries may not be known prior to surgery and some decisions may have to be taken during the surgery.
- Possible need for additional surgeries depending on the nature and extent of injury (retinal detachment surgery, keratoplasty, secondary IOL implantation, evisceration etc.).
- IOL implantation may not be possible at the first surgery and patient may need glasses or contact lens for visual rehabilitation.
- Visual prognosis may be guarded and long-term follow-ups may be required for possible late complications like secondary glaucoma/amblyopia/inflammation/visual axis opacification.

7.8 Surgical Decision-Making

Majority of the steps of pediatric cataract management post trauma are similar to the general steps discussed earlier in this book, however, there are some fine nuances which one might have to learn. Also, the surgical plan may vary depending upon the type of trauma and duration since injury. A corneal tear along with a cataract may necessitate tear repair with or without managing cataract. Similarly, an old self-sealed corneal tear with cataract may only require cataract management. Following considerations are necessary while planning surgery for a traumatic cataract.

7.8.1 Optical Correction

The use of an IOL in traumatic cataracts is well acknowledged. It offers all the benefits of refractive correction in the phakic plane, as discussed in earlier chapters [17]. It is the best modality for correction of aphakia in children that closely simulates the image formed by the normal crystalline lens. The spectacle or contact lens dependence of an appropriately corrected pseudophakic child is usually limited to reading [6].

The ideal, in bag implantation of IOL may not always be possible due to altered ocular anatomy in trauma. There may be damage to the capsular bag, zonules and iris which may make IOL implantation challenging and predispose it to decentration or pupillary capture in the post-operative period.

The guidelines related to IOL power under-correction remain the same in trauma and have been previously discussed in other chapters.

The use of contact lenses for optical rehabilitation post trauma offers an additional advantage of compensating for irregular corneal curvature caused by scarring. However, the use of contact lens in children is difficult due to associated discomfort and poor motivation. Also maintaining lens hygiene may be difficult and may lead to corneal infections.

7.8.2 Timing of Surgery

The timing of traumatic cataract surgery in children is a dilemma with no clear consensus in literature.

In open globe injuries, some authors prefer cataract management with IOL implantation as a part of primary surgery while others prefer to do it later [18–21]. We feel that there are definite advantages of the two-staged approach and the lens may be left untouched at the time of initial corneal/scleral repair even in the presence of an anterior capsular breach. Anterior capsule rupture with lens cortical matter in the anterior chamber is usually well tolerated in children. There is however a risk of lens matter-induced granulomatous inflammation (phacoanaphylactic endophthalmitis) and IOP spikes for which the physician must be watchful.

After the episode of trauma (and primary repair in open globe injuries) we prefer to medically control the ocular inflammation and IOP prior to cataract surgery, even when flocculent lens matter is present in anterior chamber. Topical steroids, cycloplegics and anti-glaucoma (aqueous suppressants) medications are the mainstay. The usual duration of pre-surgical medical management under close observation is about 2–4 weeks, after which cataract surgery with or without IOL implantation may be performed. The outcome of cataract surgery is better when the inflammation, hyphema and IOP are controlled. As discussed earlier, during the wait, it is of utmost importance to rule out associated injury to ocular structures (e.g. posterior capsule rupture, vitreous haemorrhage and retinal detachment) as some of these may warrant an earlier intervention. Similarly, medically uncontrolled IOP may also necessitate early surgery.

Cataract surgery with IOL implantation along with the primary repair of ocular trauma may be considered in young children with a clean injury and minimal collateral damage. This would prevent repeat general anaesthesia and minimize chances of amblyopia, but this decision should be taken on a case-to-case basis after a complete assessment of the extent of ocular injury. Sometimes surgical plan has to be altered on the operating table despite a comprehensive pre-operative workup.

7.8.3 Choice of Anaesthesia

General anaesthesia is preferable even in older children, who might otherwise be cooperative for local anaesthesia, to allow flexibility of the surgical plan. As the surgery may get painful (with waning effect of local anaesthesia) and prolonged (e.g. need for additional vitrectomy or placement of endocapsular ring) so general anaesthesia is advisable. Moreover, peribulbar block raises the intraocular pressure and is best avoided in patients with trauma.

Preoperatively, intravenous mannitol 1–2 g/kg over 30–60 min may be given in children with open globe injuries to reduce the vitreous volume.

7.8.4 Incision and Tunnel

The choice between corneal and scleral tunnel incision varies on a case-to-case basis. When the integrity of the capsular bag or the zonular support is doubtful, the IOL (foldable or rigid) finally implanted may differ from the initial choice. A scleral tunnel gives the flexibility to implant a rigid lens by easy wound extension if the situation requires, which may be a limitation with corneal incisions.

7.8.5 Synechiolysis

Traumatic cataracts are often associated with both anterior and posterior synechiae (Figs. 7.14 and 7.15). It is necessary to perform synechiolysis in these eyes to enable pupil dilatation and improve the visualization of the lens during surgery. A viscoelastic cannula, Sinsky hook or an iris repositor may be used for this purpose. Occlusiopupillae with no pupillary opening may occur with long-standing inflammation and this is also managed similarly (Fig. 7.16). Peroperative prophylactic peripheral iridectomy may be considered in such cases as they are more likely to redevelop posterior synechiae post-operatively.

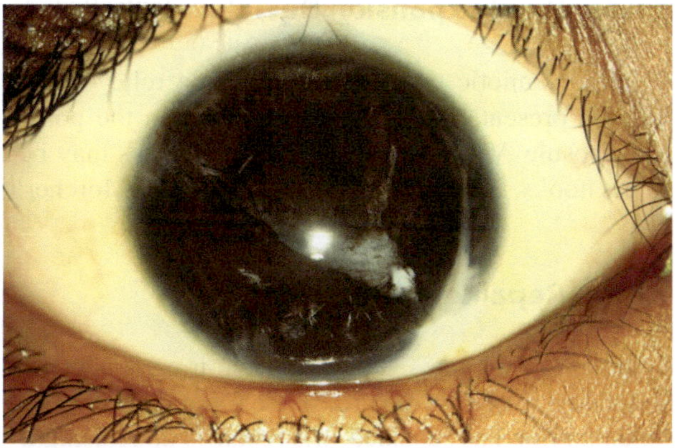

Fig. 7.14 Dense posterior synechia in late presentation after trauma

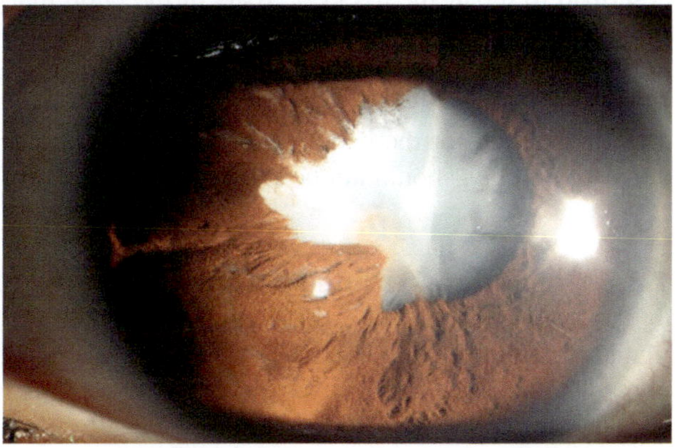

Fig. 7.15 Posterior synechia in two quadrants in early presentation after trauma

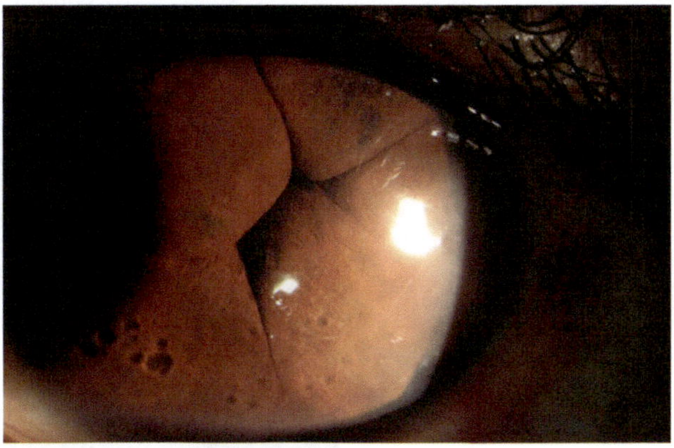

Fig. 7.16 Complete occlusion pupillae in late presentation

7.8.6 Pupil Expansion Devices

Extremely miotic or distorted pupil not relieved by synechiolysis may occur in delayed presentation with fibrosis between the posterior iris surface and anterior lens capsule. Various pupil expansion devices may be used in such situations such as iris hooks, B-hex ring, Malyugin ring and Morcher ring.

7.8.7 Repair of Iris and Pupil

Trauma to iris may present as an irregular pupil, iridodialysis or polycoria. Iridodialysis may be repaired at the time of primary surgery or later when the ocular inflammation has subsided. Iris repair is done using a series of double-armed 10-0 Prolene sutures on a long, straight STC-6 needle. Various techniques have been described to repair the iris [12]. Tears of the pupil margin alter the size, shape and reaction of the pupil resulting in glare and photophobia (Fig. 7.17). For this, a pupilloplasty procedure with 10-0 Prolene may be done at the time of initial surgery but is better performed as a secondary procedure in a non-inflamed, pseudophakic eye after accounting for the patient's symptoms and level of discomfort. These procedures, preferably, should not be attempted by beginners.

7.8.8 Anterior Capsule Management

Management of the lens capsule in traumatic cataract cases is very challenging and unpredictable, especially in eyes involving penetrating trauma. The anterior capsule may be ruptured or fibrosed and a usual capsulorhexis may not be possible in all cases (Fig. 7.18).

The decision to attempt a round regular capsulorhexis or a can-opener capsulotomy is often made during surgery after anterior capsule staining with 0.1% Trypan blue dye. A thick fibrosed capsule may resist the traditional shearing force and

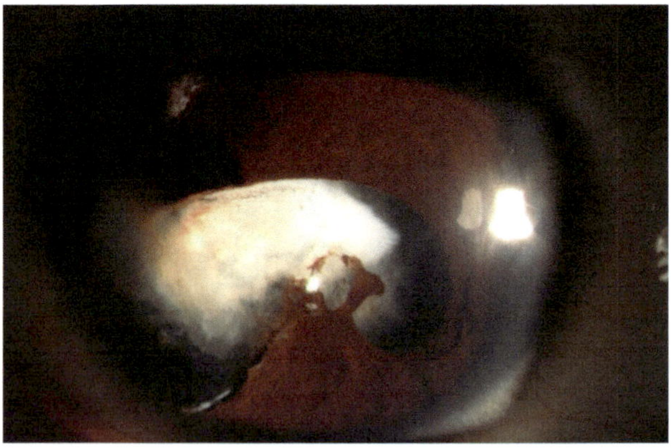

Fig. 7.17 Tear of pupillary margin with presence of synechia

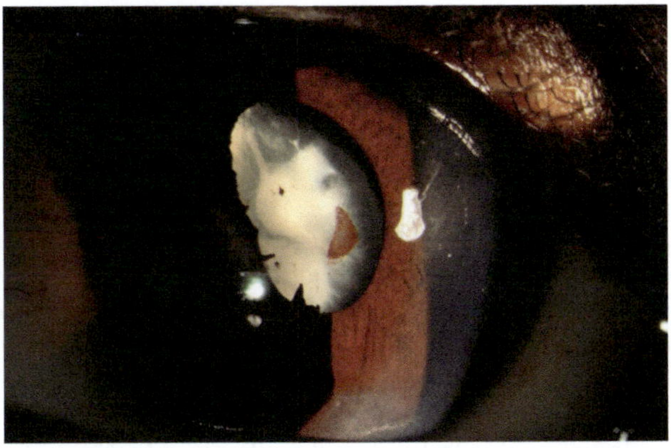

Fig. 7.18 Anterior capsular fibrotic plaque with cataractous lens

require mechanical cutting with micro scissors. A vitrector-assisted capsulotomy is also a good alternative, especially when the anterior capsule is fibrotic and scarred. The cut rate and vacuum settings need to be individualized but usually a high cut rate and low vacuum settings are preferred while dealing with the lens capsule. Other methods to handle a very dense fibrous capsule are radiofrequency diathermy and plasma blade.

7.8.9 Hydro Procedures

The integrity of the posterior lens capsule is often doubtful in traumatic cataract and hence it is better to avoid hydro procedures.

7.8.10 Nucleus Management

The nucleus and cortex are usually fluffy and can be easily removed by irrigation and aspiration. However, in few cases especially the ones with delayed presentation, the nucleus may be hardened requiring phacoemulsification or delivery. Viscoelastic or wire-vectis assisted nucleus delivery may be performed.

7.8.11 Posterior Capsule

Management of the posterior capsule depends on its integrity and the age of the patient. Inability to do a post-operative Nd:YAG laser capsulotomy is a major challenge to keep the visual axis clear in young children. Posterior capsular opacification (PCO) or visual axis opacification (VAO) is rapid in children post trauma. Performing a primary posterior capsulorhexis with or without anterior vitrectomy delays the formation and decreases the incidence of visual axis opacification (VAO). This has been discussed in detail in earlier chapters. The procedure may be performed before or after IOL implantation. In older children, visually significant PCO is managed with Nd:YAG laser capsulotomy.

7.8.12 Vitrectomy

The anterior vitreous face acts as a scaffold for lens epithelial cells causing VAO. Thus, a thorough anterior vitrectomy is mandatory especially in cases having pre-operative vitreous disturbances and in young children undergoing a primary posterior capsulotomy. Inadequate anterior vitrectomy may cause undue traction and retinal tears/detachments in the late post-operative period. Vitreous management is one of the most important steps in pediatric cataract surgery.

Initial goal is to localize the vitreous which may be incarcerated in the wound, present in the subconjunctival space or the anterior chamber. Intra cameral triamcinolone may be used to identify the vitreous in the anterior chamber and is an important tool for a thorough vitrectomy. The vitrectomy settings vary with the machine used but usually high cut rate (800–1500 cpm) and low vacuum settings (100–150 mmHg) are used. These avoid excessive vitreous traction. Vitrectomy should initially be completed at the entry/exit wound before proceeding intraocularly. Lens matter or uveal tissue may be incarcerated along with vitreous in penetrating trauma and should also be excised either manually or preferably with the vitrectomy probe. Vitrector can also be used to cut and extract thick calcified anterior lens capsule or solid lens matter in the anterior chamber. Such scenarios require a lower cut rate (150–300 cpm) with high vacuum settings (150–200 mm Hg). Care should be taken while using vitrectomy as the probe may inadvertently injure normal tissues such as the iris or intact lens capsule. Intraoperatively, retinal examination must be done.

7.8.13 Placement and Choice of Intraocular Lens

In-the-bag placement of the IOL is preferred as that is the most physiological space for the lens. This reduces chances of post-operative glaucoma, lens decentration, minimizes chances of uveitis, pupillary capture and delays PCO formation [14, 15]. In situations when the IOL is implanted in the sulcus, capturing the IOL optic through the anterior capsulorhexis ensures IOL centration and reduces the chances of its subsequent pupillary capture. Due to greater inflammation and frequent iris injury in trauma, pupillary capture of a sulcus fixated IOL is more frequent in trauma when compared to non-traumatic cases (Fig. 7.19).

IOL implantation in presence of zonulodialysis has been discussed later.

Hydrophobic acrylic or heparin surface-modified hydrophilic foldable IOLs should be implanted in the bag as a first choice. A 3 piece foldable IOL with prolene haptics may be a second choice when implanted in the sulcus. A rigid polymethylmethacrylate (PMMA) IOL is the next option. However, it is not always possible to fixate the IOL in the capsular bag or sulcus due to anterior and/or posterior capsule

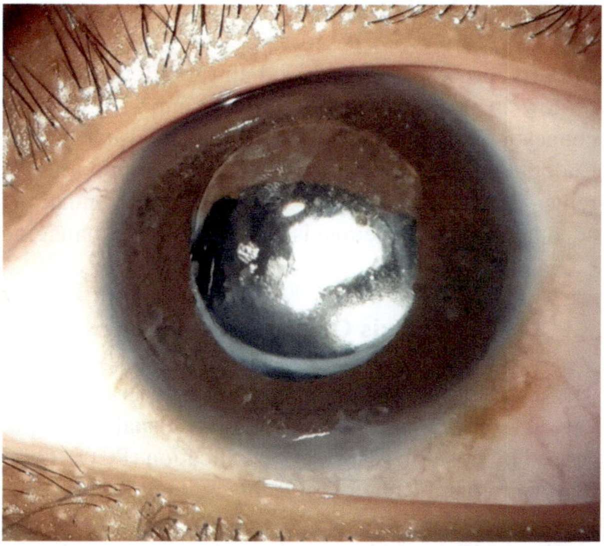

Fig. 7.19 Pupillary capture after sulcus placement of PMMA IOL

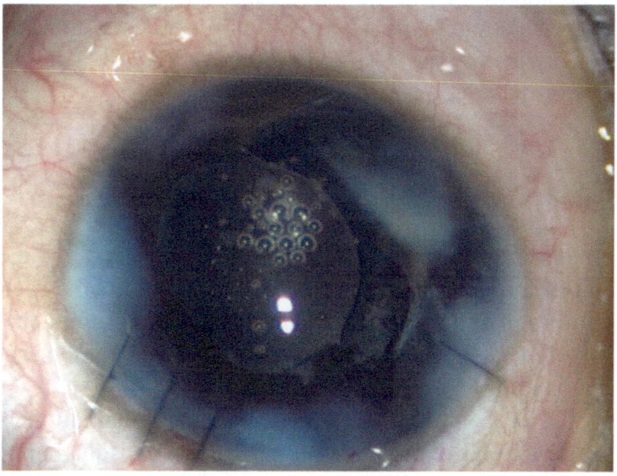

Fig. 7.20 Retro fixated iris claw lens in presence of capsular bag and iris injury

tears from trauma or an earlier surgical procedure. Anterior chamber placement, iris fixation (Fig. 7.20) and scleral anchoring (with or without sutures) of IOLs are alternatives depending on surgical expertise [16, 22–24].

7.9 Complications

Complications related to pediatric cataract surgery have been discussed in detail in the previous chapter. A few important ones are highlighted here.

7.9.1 Endophthalmitis

In early post-operative period threshold for suspecting endophthalmitis should be low in pediatric patients with trauma. Any unexplained pain, circumcorneal congestion, lid oedema or decrease in visual acuity should alert the caregiver. Endophthalmitis has been discussed in the previous chapter. However, it should be remembered that higher post-operative inflammation is common in children and adequate steroid coverage is necessary while managing traumatic cataract.

7.9.2 Visual Axis Opacification

The most important and common post-operative complication following pediatric cataract surgery following trauma is visual axis opacification (VAO) commonly caused by posterior capsular opacification (PCO). Other causes of VAO are secondary membrane formation, IOL precipitates, pupillary capture and IOL decentration or dislocation.

Use of hydrophobic acrylic IOLs and central primary posterior capsulorhexis with anterior vitrectomy decreases and delays the VAO significantly as discussed earlier. Patients with visually significant VAO and in whom Nd:YAG laser capsulotomy is not possible or not effective, require a surgical capsulotomy or membranectomy under general anaesthesia.

7.9.3 IOL Capture and Decentration

As discussed earlier in the book appropriately sized capsulorhexes, in-the-bag IOL implantation and optic capture of IOL are some techniques used to ensure IOL centration and prevent its pupillary capture. Optic capture of a 3 piece sulcus fixated IOL also achieves the same. However, these surgical steps may be extremely challenging in eyes with trauma.

IOL decentration may occur when implantation is done in presence of traumatic zonular dialysis and/or inadequate capsular support. When the zonulodialysis involves about 3 clock hours carefully aspirating the cataract and placing a 3 piece foldable or a rigid IOL in the bag with placement of haptics in the meridian of the area of dehiscence, spreads out the bag keeping the IOL centred. Minimal manipulation of the IOL should be done after placement in the bag to prevent extension of zonular damage. Placement of endocapsular ring or capsular tension ring (ECR/CTR) along with in-the-bag placement of IOL may also be helpful in the presence of zonular disruption. In cases where zonulodialysis noted intraoperatively is less than 6 clock hours, a simple ECR may be sufficient. However, eyes with more than 180° of zonulodialysis require sutured ring segments or Cionni ring. Endo capsular rings or segments are not recommended in cases with posterior capsular dehiscence. Sectoral iris and capsular bag fibrosis may cause IOL placement partially in the bag and partially in the sulcus. This should be avoided as it may also lead to decentration

(Fig. 7.21). With the gradual contraction of the capsular bag, the initially subtle tilt of IOL may increase, causing significant lenticular astigmatism. Significant decentration or dislocation may require IOL repositioning or explantation (Fig. 7.22).

7.9.4 Amblyopia

Management of amblyopia is a major challenge with any pediatric cataract surgery as discussed at several places in this book. Amblyopia can develop prior to surgery in delayed presentation or due to delay between primary repair and definitive cataract management. Factors such as VAO, decentration of IOL, uncorrected residual refractive error, irregular astigmatism and loss of accommodation contribute post-operatively to development of amblyopia. Poor compliance to use of glasses (or contact lens) and occlusion in the post-operative period are major challenges.

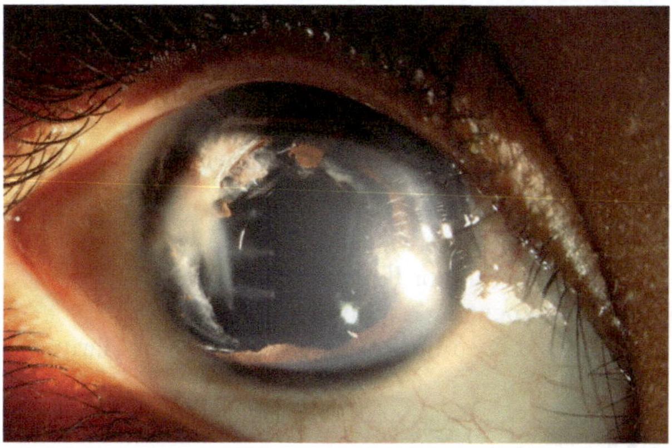

Fig. 7.21 Tilting and decentration of IOL due to fibrosis and anterior synechia

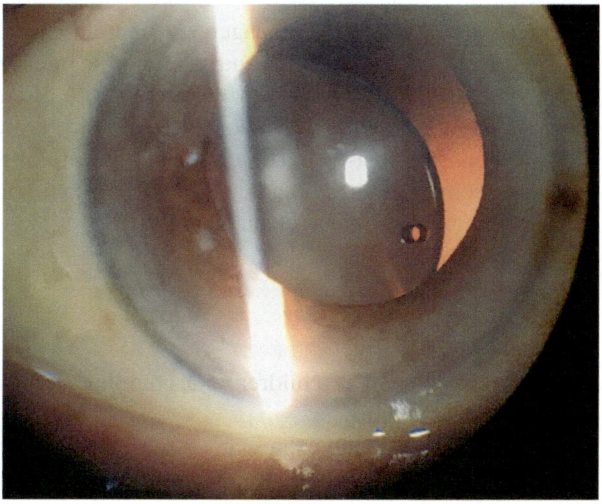

Fig. 7.22 Significant decentration requires repositioning or explantation (Photo courtesy: Dr. Vikas Chahal, Lucknow, India)

Following a successful surgical outcome, the parents of young children should be counselled about strict compliance to amblyopia therapy to get maximum visual benefit. This has been discussed in detail in the next chapter.

7.10 Follow-Up Examinations

The children should be remain admitted for 2–3 days following the surgery. Serial follow-up and examinations under anaesthesia (for uncooperative children) are required in post-operative period. Following discharge, follow-ups should be initially at weekly and subsequently at monthly intervals (Table 6.3). Follow-up examinations should include assessment of visual acuity, refraction, subjective improvement, ocular alignment, detection and management of amblyopia. Slit lamp examination, assessment of VAO, fundus evaluation and IOP assessment should also be carried out at each visit. A scan for changes in axial length and trial of contact lenses for corneal astigmatism may be done when indicated.

Corneal sutures placed at the time of primary surgery may be removed at 4–6 weeks if they are loose, causing astigmatism or foreign body sensation. Wound integrity using fluorescein dye (Seidel test) should be performed prior to suture removal.

"REAL" is an acronym to remember the points to be addressed in pediatric cataract follow-ups.

R: Refraction and visual acuity
E: Eye pressure or IOP
A: Alignment and amblyopia
L: Lens related factors such as visual axis clarity

7.11 Prognosis

Prognosis after successful management of traumatic cataract depends on associated injuries. Corneal scarring and posterior segment involvement are commonly responsible for adverse outcomes. About 50–75% of children achieve a final visual acuity of 20/60 or better and about 20% require more than one surgery [5, 25]. Mild-to-moderate post-operative complications are observed in about 15% of children and secondary glaucoma development is common in eyes with blunt trauma undergoing traumatic cataract surgery [26].

7.12 Summary

- Traumatic cataract in children is a complex situation and challenges even the skilled ophthalmologist.
- Comprehensive ocular examination, relevant investigations, careful planning and prognostication of each patient with respect to timing and nature of surgery are essential.

- A gap of 2–4 weeks after primary repair is preferable for resolution of ocular inflammation before cataract surgery. Topical steroids, cycloplegics and anti-glaucoma treatment may be needed during this time.
- An unnecessary delay in definitive treatment must be avoided during the critical age for the development of amblyopia (till about 6 years).
- IOLs should be implanted in children with traumatic cataract whenever possible.
- A close, long-term follow-up is required which may include multiple examinations under anaesthesia.
- Counselling of parents is critical for good clinical outcome and satisfaction. The need for serial follow-ups, importance of post-operative glasses, occlusion and possibility of multiple surgeries should be clearly explained.

Multiple Choice Questions

1. The following are true about blunt trauma on the lens:
   (a) Vossius ring is the main reason for reduced visual acuity.
   (b) Vossius ring is a permanent sign.
   (c) Traumatic cataract secondary to blunt trauma is usually rosette shaped.
   (d) Anterior cortex is the most commonly involved area in the lens.

   Answer: *(c) Traumatic cataract secondary to blunt trauma is usually rosette shaped.* Vossius ring is the imprinting of iris pigments on the anterior lens capsule post injury. They are unlikely to be present in the central visual axis, hence are visually insignificant and may also fade away over a period of time.

2. The intraocular lens of choice in a case of pediatric traumatic cataract with a ruptured posterior lens capsule and intact capsulorhexis is:
   (a) PMMA lens.
   (b) Single-piece acrylic lens.
   (c) Three-piece acrylic lens.
   (d) Scleral fixated intraocular lens.

   Answer: *(c) Three-piece acrylic lens.* In cases of trauma presenting with pre-existing damage to posterior lens capsule, when IOL cannot be placed in the bag safely, the best option would be to place a three-piece acrylic IOL in the sulcus provided there is good anterior capsular support.

3. The follow-up of a case of traumatic cataract with angle recession post-cataract extraction and IOL implantation in a 1-year-old child should include all of the following except:
   (a) Horizontal corneal diameter
   (b) Refraction
   (c) Intraocular pressure
   (d) Keratometry reading

   Answer: *(d) Keratometry reading.* In cases of traumatic cataract and angle recession, monitoring of intraocular pressure and Horizontal corneal diameter is of utmost importance. Refraction is a must during follow-up of pediatric cataract cases to look for myopic shift and to give appropriate glasses/contact lens.

4. Which of the following is an inert intraocular foreign body?
   (a) Iron
   (b) Copper
   (c) Stone
   (d) Wood

   Answer: *(c) Stone*. Iron and Copper being metals generate reactions while inside the eye. Wood behaves as a vegetative matter. A stone particle, especially during chipping process comes as a projectile at high speed and temperature, thus behaving as a relatively inert foreign body.

5. Which of the following are useful investigative modalities for localizing intraocular foreign body of unknown origin except?
   (a) CT scan
   (b) X-Ray
   (c) MRI scan
   (d) Ultrasonography

   Answer: *(c) MRI scan*. When the nature of intraocular foreign body is unknown, an MRI is contra-indicated as any metallic foreign body may change position and cause further damage to ocular structures due to the magnetic field.

6. Which among the following is a type of closed globe injury?
   (a) Laceration
   (b) Penetration
   (c) Contusion
   (d) IOFB (intraocular foreign body)

   Answer: *(c) Contusion*. Laceration, penetration and IOFB are types of open globe injuries whereas contusion and lamellar laceration are closed globe injuries.

References

1. Eckstein M, Vijayalakshmi P, Killedar M, et al. Aetiology of childhood cataract in South India. Br J Ophthalmol. 1996;80:628–32.
2. Reddy AK, Ray R, Yen YG. Surgical intervention of traumatic cataracts in children: epidemiology, complications and outcomes. J AAPOS. 2009;13:170–4.
3. Johar SR, Savalia NK, Vasavada AR, Gupta PD. Epidemiology based etiological study of pediatric cataract in western India. Indian J Med Sci. 2004;58:115–21.
4. Du Y, He W, Sun X, et al. Traumatic cataract in children in eastern China: Shanghai Pediatric Cataract Study. Sci Rep. 2018;8:2588. https://doi.org/10.1038/s41598-018-20982-1.

5. Krishnamachary M, Rathi V, Gupta S. Management of traumatic cataract in children. J Cataract Refract Surg. 1997;23(Suppl 1):681–7. https://doi.org/10.1016/s0886-3350(97)80054-5.
6. von Noorden GK, Crawford MLJ. The sensitive period. Trans Ophthalmol Soc UK. 1979;99:442–6.
7. Taylor D. Monocular infantile cataract, intraocular lenses and amblyopia (editorial). Br J Ophthalmol. 1989;73:857–8.
8. Lambert SR, Drack AV. Infantile cataracts. Surv Ophthalmol. 1996;40:427–58.
9. Dutton JJ, Baker JD, Hiles DA, Morgan KS. Visual rehabilitation of aphakic children. Surv Ophthalmol. 1990;34:365–84.
10. Alfaro DV, Jablon EP, Rodriguez Fontal M, et al. Fishing- related ocular trauma. Am J Ophthalmol. 2005;139:488–92.
11. Kuhn F, Morris R, Witherspoon CD, Mester V. The Birmingham Eye Trauma Terminology system (BETT). J Fr Ophtalmol. 2004;27(2):206–10.
12. Kuhn F, Morris R, Witherspoon CD, et al. A standardized classification of ocular trauma. Ophthalmology. 1996;103:240–3.
13. Ben Ezra D, Cohen E, Rose L. Traumatic cataract in children: correction of aphakia by contact lens or intraocular lens. Am J Ophthalmol. 1997;123:773–82.
14. Kothari M, Bhaskare A, Mete D, Toshniwal S, Doshi P, Kaul S. Evaluation of central, steady, maintained fixation grading for predicting inter-eye visual acuity difference to diagnose and treat amblyopia in strabismic patients. Indian J Ophthalmol. 2009;57:281–4.
15. Deramo VA, Shah GK, Baumal CR, Fineman MS, Corrěa ZM, Benson WE, et al. The role of ultrasound biomicroscopy in ocular trauma. Trans Am Ophthalmol Soc. 1998;96:355–65.
16. Tabatabaei SA, Rajabi MB, Tabatabaei SM, Soleimani S, Rahimi F, Yaseri M. Early versus late traumatic cataract surgery and intraocular lens implantation. Eye (Lond). 2017;31(8):1199–204.
17. Agrawal S, Singh V, Yadav A, Katiyar V. Orthoptic relevance of refractive correction in the phakic plane in unilateral high refractive errors in adults. Oman J Ophthalmol. 2016;9:196–8.
18. Hoffman RS, Fine IH, Packer M. Scleral fixation without conjunctival dissection. J Cataract Refract Surg. 2006;32:1907–12.
19. Pandey SK, Ram J, Werner L, et al. Visual results and postoperative complications of capsular bag and ciliary sulcus fixation of posterior chamber intraocular lenses in children with traumatic cataracts. J Cataract Refract Surg. 1999;25:1576–84.
20. Ram J, Pandey SK, Apple DJ, et al. Effect of in-the-bag intraocular lens fixation on the prevention of posterior capsule opacification. J Cataract Refract Surg. 2001;27:1039–46.
21. Kumar DA, Agarwal A, Prakash D, et al. Glued intrascleral fixation of posterior chamber intraocular lens in children. Am J Ophthalmol. 2012;153:594–601. 601.e591–601.e592
22. Donaldson KE, Gorscak JJ, Budenz DL, Feuer WJ, Benz MS, Forster RK. Anterior chamber and sutured posterior chamber intraocular lenses in eyes with poor capsular support. J Cataract Refract Surg. 2005;31:903–9.
23. Baykara M, Ozcetin H, Yilmaz S, Timuçin OB. Posterior iris fixation of the iris-claw intraocular lens implantation through a scleral tunnel incision. Am J Ophthalmol. 2007;144:586–91.
24. Sen P, S VK, Bhende P, Rishi P, Rishi E, Rao C, et al. Surgical outcomes and complications of sutured scleral fixated intraocular lenses in pediatric eyes. Can J Ophthalmol. 2018;53:49–55.
25. Gogate P, Sahasrabudhe M, Shah M, Patil S, Kulkarni A. Causes, epidemiology, and long-term outcome of traumatic cataracts in children in rural India. Indian J Ophthalmol. 2012;60:481–6.
26. Blum M, Tetz MR, Greiner C, Voelcker HE. Treatment of traumatic cataracts. J Cataract Refract Surg. 1996;22(3):342–6.

Post-operative Rehabilitation After Cataract Surgery in Children

8

Soveeta Rath, Suma Ganesh, and Rolli Khurana

8.1 Introduction

Successful management of pediatric cataract depends on optimal visual rehabilitation after cataract surgery. Early and appropriate refractive correction after cataract surgery is crucial to avoid amblyopia and facilitate good visual outcomes. This crucial step mandates regular post-operative follow-up with detailed evaluation at every visit. Equally important is timely management of abnormalities related to intraocular pressure (IOP), clarity of visual axis, ocular alignment, retina and optic disc. Cataract surgery alone, without regular post-operative follow-ups and rehabilitation may have outcomes similar to an unoperated child.

This chapter primarily covers visual rehabilitation after cataract surgery in children.

8.2 Post-operative Follow-Ups

Before the surgery, parents must be explained that without timely and long-term follow-up visits, the efforts put in by the medical team as well as the parents may become futile. As has been discussed in earlier chapters, after discharge the children should be examined every week for a month. Thereafter, 3 monthly follow-ups are essential for 6 months, followed by 6 monthly reviews till 8 years of age. Subsequently, the children should be seen annually till the refraction stabilises. In

S. Rath (✉) · S. Ganesh
Dr Shroff's Charity Eye Hospital, Delhi, India

R. Khurana
Eye Department, Armed Forces Medical Services, Military Hospital, Ahmedabad, Gujarat, India

S. Agrawal (ed.), *Pediatric Cataract*,
https://doi.org/10.1007/978-981-16-1736-2_8

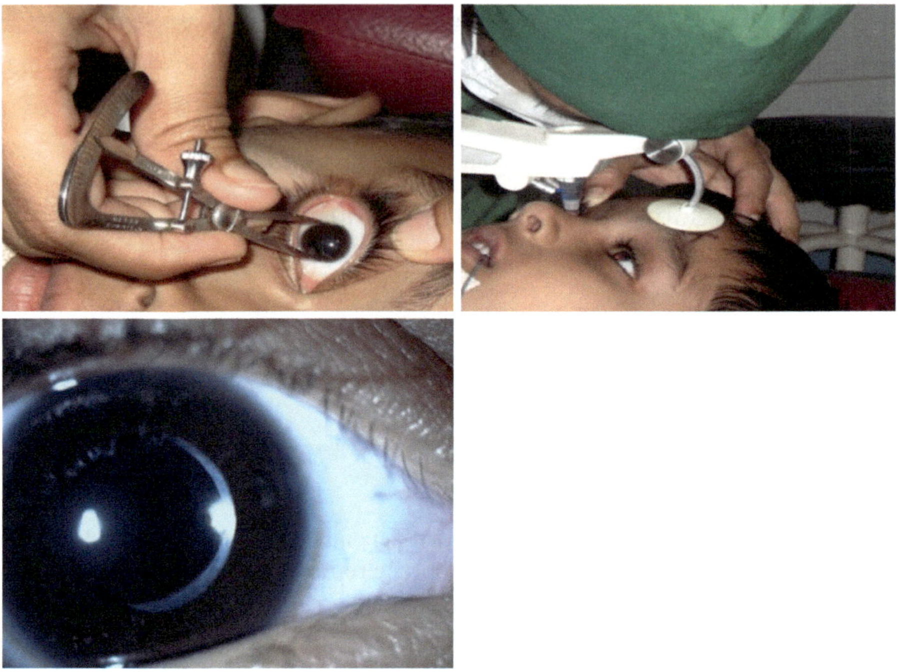

Fig. 8.1 Measurement of corneal diameter, intraocular pressure and anterior segment examination during examination under anaesthesia

order to ensure comprehensive assessment, periodic examinations under anaesthesia (EUA) should be considered in children younger than 4 years (Fig. 8.1).

Every follow-up examination after cataract surgery may need a customised approach depending upon the time since surgery. Special focus may be needed to assess wound integrity, sutures, IOL position and inflammation in the immediate post-operative period. Visual acuity assessment, refraction, IOP and media clarity evaluation are important during the later follow-up visits. Overall, the key focus during follow-up examination is to assess vision and binocular interaction in children and, to identify any potential amblyogenic factor. Table 8.1 highlights some of the key concerns and their assessment during the follow-up period.

8.3 Optical Rehabilitation

The goal of visual rehabilitation following cataract surgery is attained only after accurate refraction and spectacle prescription. With loss of accommodation post-operatively, these children essentially need glasses for near work. However, most of them also need correction for distance depending on the age and under-correction of IOL power.

Table 8.1 Issues to be addressed and examination required during follow-ups

Changing refractive errors • Visual acuity • Refraction • Improvement
Visual axis opacification • Distant direct ophthalmoscopy • Slit lamp examination
Amblyopia • Best corrected visual acuity • Near vision • Contrast
Strabismus • Orthoptic checkup
Glaucoma • IOP • Corneal diameter • Optic disc • Axial Length
Retinal breaks/detachment • Indirect ophthalmoscopy

8.3.1 Visual Acuity Assessment and Refraction

Assessing the visual acuity in a child is foremost step prior to performing refraction. Efforts must be made using age appropriate methods to have an objective estimate of existing visual acuity in children [1]. Parents of preschool children must be encouraged to teach their children at home, the responses to 'E' chart to enable accurate visual acuity assessment at clinics. Evaluation for subjective improvement in vision post refraction is a recommended step wherever possible to fine tune optical prescription.

Refraction should preferably be performed after the surgery of the first eye to decide on any adjustment of intraocular lens power to be implanted in the other eye. While aphakic children are given a temporary correction at the time of discharge, they should undergo refraction within 2 weeks of surgery with prescription of appropriate glasses or contact lens [2]. In pseudophakic children refraction should be performed at about 1 month post-operatively. It should be repeated after suture removal (usually done at 6 weeks, if required) in all children before final prescription of glasses. Retinoscopy should be performed after mydriasis, although no cycloplegia is needed.

With patience, refraction can be accurately done is most children. However, those who are uncooperative or in whom suture removal is planned, the procedure may be performed under anaesthesia following suture removal.

Refractive status of the eye is subject to change due to the continuous growth of the eyeball. Thus, a periodic refraction is necessary. A disproportionate myopic shift with respect to axial length hints towards secondary glaucoma [3–5].

8.3.2 Optical Correction

Early optical rehabilitation stimulates binocularity with reduction in the incidence of amblyopia and strabismus. While in the bag IOL implantation aiming emmetropia would have been ideal, dynamic nature of the visual system in children makes IOL implantation in very young children tricky with possibilities of refractive surprises and related complications. With the removal of natural crystalline lens, loss of accommodation is the major concern warranting correction for all distances. Furthermore, residual refractive error for correction would vary depending upon the phakic status of a child and would require a customised approach. The need for near correction and its amount is based on the proximity of area of visual interest at different ages, as discussed in the next section.

8.3.2.1 Pseudophakic Children

After primary implantation of IOL with planned under-correction nearly all infants have amblyogenic residual hyperopia. Pseudophakic children should be prescribed the entire spherical and cylindrical power calculated on a dilated retinoscopy. After compensating for the working distance (usually between 1.0 and 2.0 D) based on the retinoscopy, the prescription is finalised with near addition of +2.00 to +3.00 Dioptres Sphere (DS).

In children up to 2 years of age only near correction is prescribed to ensure clear vision for near activities in the absence of accommodation. This suffices as the area of interest at this age is limited to a few feet from the face. Thereafter, preschool children are corrected only for distance as their focus of attention shifts to distant objects but they are too young for bifocals. Schoolgoing children require bifocals with near addition of +2.50 to 3.00 DS according to visual demands. Executive bifocals are preferred with bisecting axis coinciding with the lower pupillary margin (Fig. 8.2). Progressive lenses are recommended for older children (Table 8.2).

Ideally, all glasses in children should be made with polycarbonate material. It is not only shatter-resistant but also has an inherent property of Ultra Violet (UV) radiation protection [6]. UV protection in pseudophakics is important since the natural protection of the crystalline lens is lost with surgery.

Children tamper and play with their glasses. It is important to use plastic flexible frames, which have lesser chances to break when handled carelessly. Also, the size of the frame should be large enough to completely cover the eyes since children

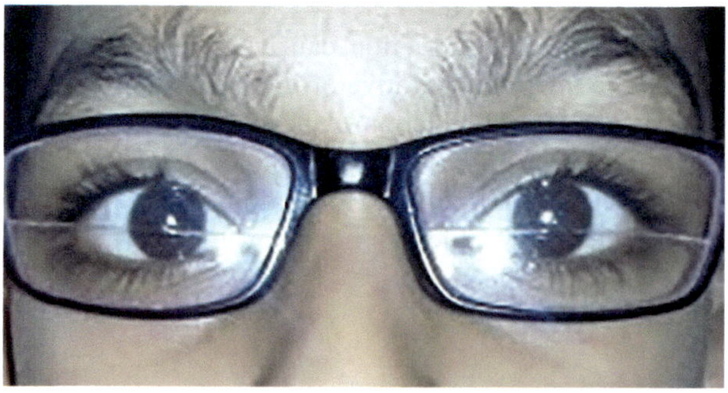

Fig. 8.2 Executive bifocals with bisecting axis coinciding with lower pupillary margin

Table 8.2 Spectacle prescription (D = Dioptres)

Pseudophakia
• Upto 2 years Only near glasses with near addition of 2 to 3 D
• Preschool (2–3 years) Only distance glasses
• School going (above 3 years) Bifocals with near addition of 2.5 to 3 D
• Adolescent (10 years and above) Progressive glasses
Aphakia
• Up to 3 years Only near glasses with near addition (over distance aphakic correction) as follows <1 year +3 D 1–2 years +2 D 2–3 years +1 D
• Above 3 years Bifocals or separate glasses for distance and near

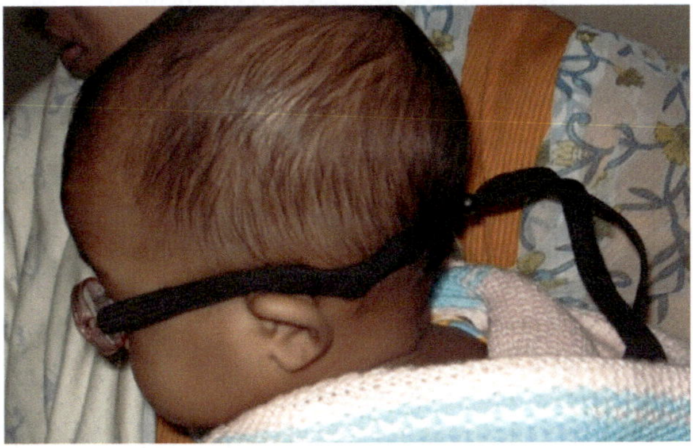

Fig. 8.3 Headbands improve compliance

tend to peep from over the glasses. Thus, smaller-sized frames may give a false impression of visual rehabilitation without actually being of any use. Moreover, compliance with glasses is another major issue. The use of headbands to fix the glasses is a useful trick (Fig. 8.3).

Contact lens is a viable option in aphakic children. However, compliance, maintenance of contact lens hygiene and eye care while using the lens remains a major issue. The use of contact lenses has been elaborated later.

8.3.2.2 Aphakic Children

During the past decade, the optical correction of aphakia in children has improved significantly. Unilateral or bilateral aphakia needs external visual rehabilitation in the form of glasses or contact lens.

As discussed earlier in the book, primary implantation of IOL remains controversial in children below 6 months of age. Children with bilateral aphakia should be definitely prescribed glasses within the first 2 weeks following surgery (and preferably at

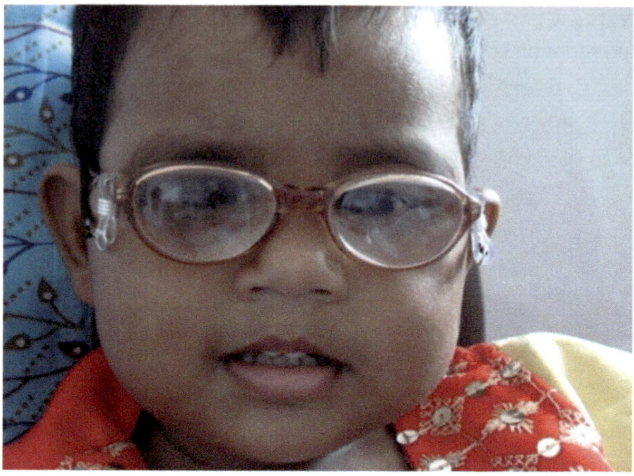

Fig. 8.4 Aphakic glasses

discharge from the hospital) in order to maximise the process of visual development. Aphakic glasses are an efficient method for visual rehabilitation in children up to 3 years of age [7]. Separate glasses for distance or an addition of bifocal segment is needed in children above 3 years of age. The major benefits of glasses in aphakic children are that they are easily available, safe, inexpensive and can be frequently changed as the eye grows. Their disadvantages include their weight, visual field narrowing, aneisokonia of about 30%, image distortion and prismatic aberrations. However, aphakic glasses are typically well tolerated by children. Being convex, these lenses are thick in centre and cause significant magnification (Fig. 8.4).

In infants and toddlers up to about 2 years of age, it is satisfactory to use single vision lenses with the focal point at about 50–66 cm. While dispensing glasses, appropriate frame size and proper centration of lenses should be ensured. Improper glasses have poor compliance as they are uncomfortable and have significant prismatic effect. They may also cause injury.

The specifications for spectacle prescription in aphakic children are as mentioned in Table 8.2. For example, if aphakic refraction at 1 m distance in a 6-month old is +22.0 D, corrected refraction would be +21.0 D and the prescription would be +24.0 D after addition of +3.0 D according to Table 8.2. If aphakic contact lenses are used, the prescription is given after calculations based on the vertex distance of the loose lens or phoropter being used for the refraction. In the above example, contact lenses of +31D would be prescribed.

Older children (>3 years of age) have greater visual demands and benefit from a traditional bifocal glasses. However, heavyweight of these glasses is a disadvantage. As discussed earlier, flat-top lower segments (executive style) are preferred as they have larger optical zones and cause lesser image jump.

In unilateral aphakia, spectacles prevent binocular vision due to significant aniseikonia and contact lenses are the obvious choice. To prevent amblyopia, spectacles (with occlusion of phakic eye) should be used only in the interim till refractive correction close to phakic plane can be restored.

Contact lens can be used in all age groups for pediatric aphakia. In unilateral cases, their use may be successfully initiated within 3 weeks of surgery (Fig. 8.5).

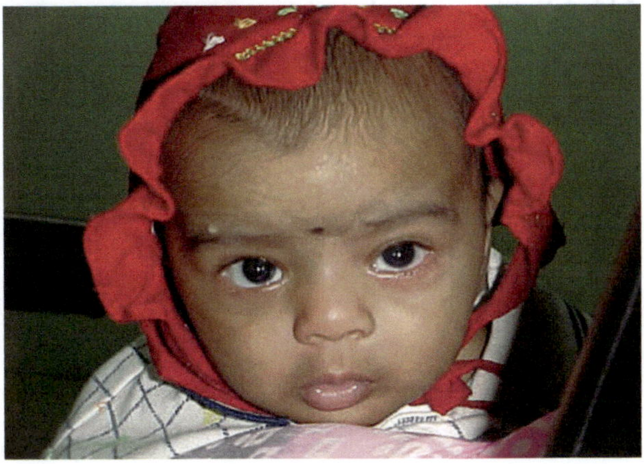

Fig. 8.5 Infant comfortable with contact lens in the left eye

Table 8.3 Advantages and disadvantages of contact lens use in children

Advantages
• Power can be adjusted easily
• Relatively safe
• 5–9% magnification
• Better field of vision
Disadvantages
• Noncompliance
• Difficulty in handling
• Frequency of lens loss
• Poor hygiene-corneal complications
• Costly

In bilateral aphakia, along with the use of contact lenses additional correction for near is prescribed as single vision glasses in infants and as bifocals in toddlers [8, 9]. The advantages and disadvantages of contact lens use have been enumerated in Table 8.3.

Contact lenses are usually well tolerated, and the power can be changed until definitive optical correction by IOL implantation is done. The Infant Aphakia Treatment Study (IATS) comparing outcomes of contact lens and IOL correction showed no significant difference in median visual acuity between two groups at 5 years, but showed more complications in the IOL group [10]. However, the results of the study must be interpreted with the understanding that the compliance of the contact lenses is limited in the developing countries, unlike the study group. This has been discussed in earlier chapters.

The available options for contact lenses in decreasing order of preference are

1. Rigid gas permeable (RGP) lenses.
2. Hydrogel lenses.
3. Silicon elastomer lenses.

The merits and demerits of each are listed in Table 8.4.

Table 8.4 Advantages and disadvantages of different types of contact lenses [7, 9]

Advantages
- Rigid gas permeable
  - Can correct high corneal astigmatism
  - Can be customised for desired power and base curve
- Hydrogel
  - Low cost
- Silicone Elastomer
  - Extended wear

Disadvantages
- Rigid gas permeable
  - Extended wear not possible
  - Frequently misplaced
- Hydrogel
  - Not recommended before 4 years of age
- Silicone Elastomer
  - Corneal and conjunctival complications
  - Poor availability

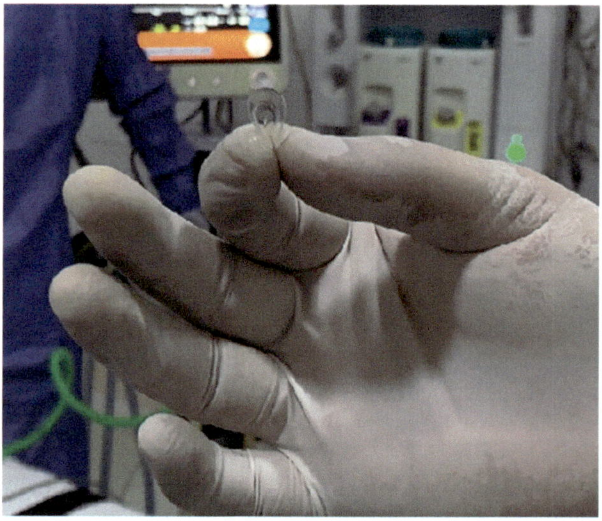

Fig. 8.6 Correct method of holding a contact lens before insertion

RGP lenses are the safest for the small developing eye. They require simple daily care which is convenient for the parents. Trial of fitting of contact lens should preferably be done under sedation or general anaesthesia based on 3 parameters—refractive error, corneal curvature and corneal diameter. Appropriate power is determined after an over-refraction under anaesthesia [7, 8].

Figures 8.6 and 8.7 demonstrate fitting of contact lens under sedation.

Though, contact lenses are a preferred over glasses in aphakic children, parental education is critical for successful outcomes. Major concerns to be addressed are poor compliance, loss of lenses, ocular irritation and hygiene.

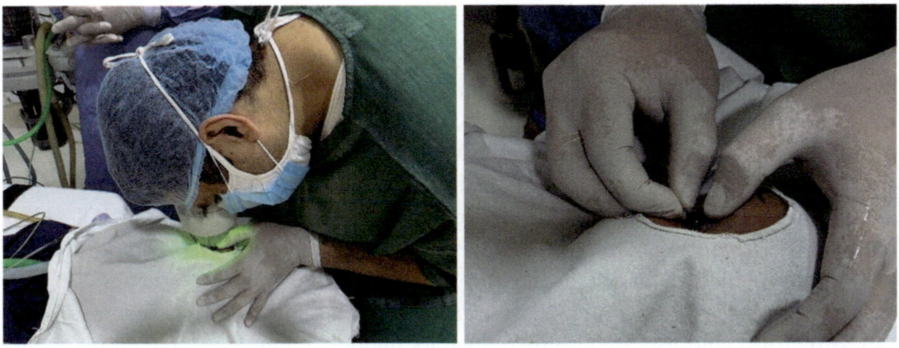

Fig. 8.7 Keratometry prior to prescription (left) and contact lens trial under anaesthesia (right)

The use of intraocular lens (IOL) implants for aphakia during childhood is the most acceptable means for visual rehabilitation. However, the timing of implantation and appropriate power calculation of the IOL is crucial. Based on the results of the IATS, early IOL placement is associated with an increased risk of having a second (or more) procedure for visual axis opacification, in order to gain at least as good of a visual outcome as compared to contact lenses, provided compliance with contact lenses can be ensured [9]. As has been detailed in earlier chapters, all children above the age of 6 months in the absence of any other ocular morbidity should undergo a primary IOL implantation at the time of cataract surgery.

When children are initially left aphakic, secondary IOL implantation is usually performed after 2 years of age, since maximum growth of the eyeball and changes in corneal curvatures have occurred by then [11, 12]. A thorough evaluation of anterior chamber, sulcus, capsular rim, posterior synechiae and vitreous prolapse is necessary before planning surgery.

The different options of IOLs, their placement, biometry and suggested under-corrections have been detailed in Chaps. 3 and 4. Suffices here to repeat that in the bag placement of foldable hydrophobic acrylic lens is preferable, biometry should be carefully performed and under-correction appropriate for age be done. Taking the mean of several biometry readings reduces the error [13]. Under-correction closer to emmetropia (lesser under-correction) is desirable in unilateral aphakia and in older children [5, 14, 15].

Following secondary IOL implantation, there are less chances of prediction errors as children are older, have longer axial length, allow accurate biometry and lesser subsequent myopic shift occurs. However, at times, secondary glaucoma causes an unexpected myopic shift and these eyes should undergo assessment for changes in axial length, IOP, optic disc, corneal diameter and corneal thickness [2, 3].

Anticipation of myopic shift, and its appropriate correction or compensation, helps achieve better functional outcomes in young eyes undergoing cataract surgery.

8.4 Visual Axis Opacification

Visual axis opacification (VAO) is synonymous to posterior capsular opacification in adults. (Fig. 8.8) This term is preferred, as in children, membranes other than the posterior capsule may also opacify. VAO occurs in 30–40% cases of pediatric cataract even after a primary posterior capsulorrhexis, the rate being higher in younger age groups [16]. Smaller capsulotomy openings, sulcus implantation of IOL, traumatic cataract and excessive intraocular inflammation are other predisposing factors. Though, multiple measures like implantation of hydrophobic or heparin-coated square edge IOLs in the bag, posterior capsulorhexis, posterior optic capture, anterior vitrectomy and use of steroids reduce its incidence yet, VAO inevitably occurs in few cases [17, 18]. Even if, on distant direct ophthalmoscopy the VAO does not appear dense, it hampers the image quality being perceived thereby having an amblyogenic effect. Hence, a thorough evaluation should be done on every follow-up to exclude the presence of VAO. The membrane formed in children is more fibrotic (Fig. 8.9) and thick as compared to adults since there is more anterior segment inflammation with rapid proliferation of lens epithelial cells in them.

In children cooperative for slit lamp evaluation and Nd:YAG laser, an attempt to perform a acapsulotomy should be done under cover of topical steroids and pressure lowering medications (Fig. 8.10). Surgical membranectomy is the procedure of choice for VAO in all other cases, that is, younger children not cooperative for YAG laser or in cases where the membrane is too fibrotic to yield on YAG laser (Fig. 8.11). Membranectomy through the pars plana route is usually performed. However, anterior limbal approach for membranectomy also shows favourable results in cases where early intervention is planned within 3–4 months of primary surgery, before excessive fibrosis occurs and adhesions form [2].

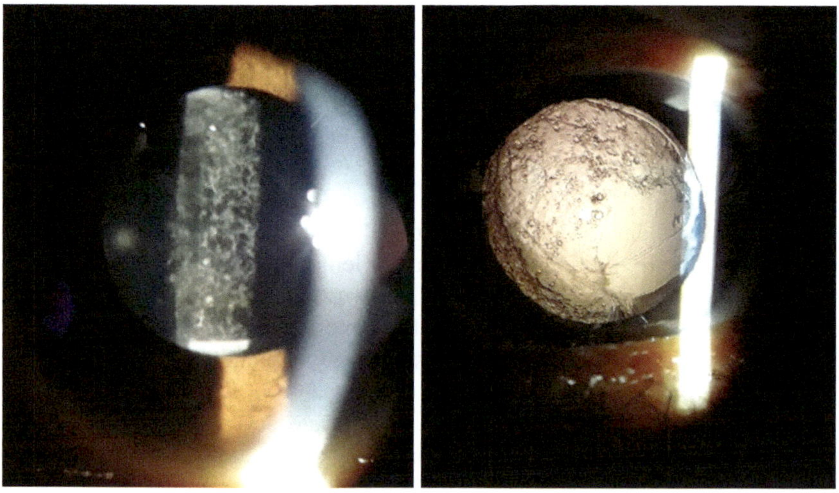

Fig. 8.8 Slit views of opacification of posterior capsule obscuring the visual axis

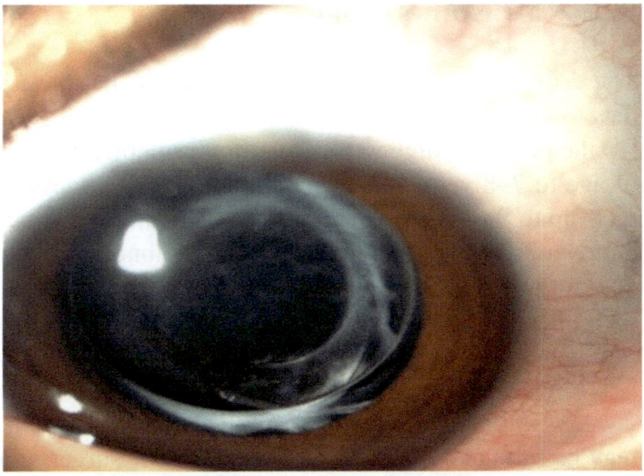

Fig. 8.9 Dense capsular membrane in a 3-year-old pseudophakic child

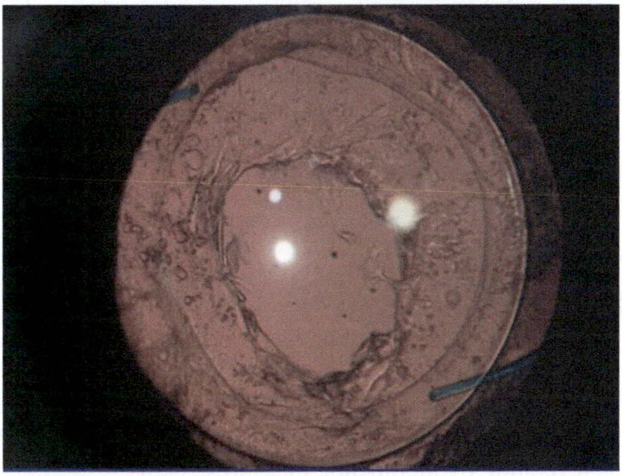

Fig. 8.10 YAG capsulotomy is successful in older and cooperative children

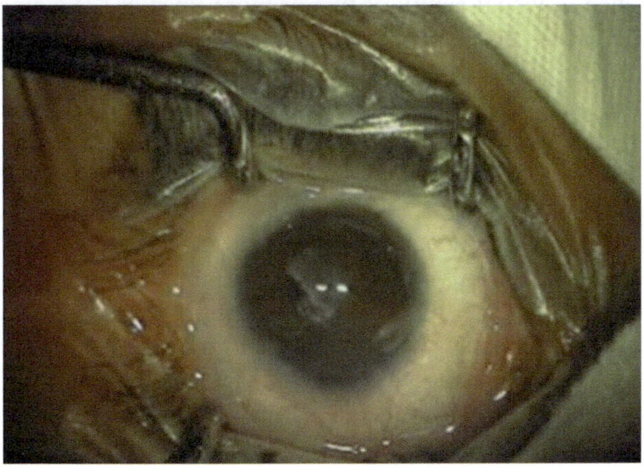

Fig. 8.11 Surgical membranectomy is indicated in non-dilating pupil and for dense membranes

8.5 Anisometropia

The critical periods in visual development that have been determined are, (i) the development of visual acuity from 20/200 to 20/20 between birth and 2–3 years, and (ii) the period of highest risk of stimulus deprivation amblyopia from a few months of age to 7–8 years [19]. Unilateral congenital, developmental and traumatic cataracts up to 8 years of age have significant amblyogenic potential. Not only stimulus deprivation induces amblyopia here, but abnormal binocular interaction due to unilaterality and anisometropia area also contributory [20]. Unilateral congenital cataracts hence require early surgical removal preferably with intraocular lens implantation. The amount of anisometropia is more when the eye is left aphakic [21]. In these children spectacles should be prescribed at discharge or latest by 2 weeks after surgery with part-time occlusion of the better eye. Contact lens usage may be initiated as early as 2–3 weeks after surgery. In unilateral pseudophake the residual hyperopia, based on age, is still amblyogenic. This anisometropia needs prompt glass prescription either as single vision or bifocals and aggressive occlusion (patching) therapy. Compliance with occlusion is a major concern and parents should be thoroughly counselled regarding this aspect in order to maximise the potential for good vision. As already discussed it is also advisable to reduce undercorrection in unilateral patients and to target near emmetropia where poor compliance is expected.

8.6 Amblyopia

Amblyopia has been defined as "decrease of visual acuity in one eye when caused by abnormal binocular interaction or occurring in one or both eyes as a result of pattern vision deprivation during visual immaturity, for which no cause can be detected during physical examination of the eye(s) and which in appropriate cases is reversible by therapeutic measures" [22].

In simple words in the absence of any detectable cause (1) an interocular difference in visual acuity of two or more lines or (2) a single eye best corrected visual acuity lesser than 6/12 or 20/40 can be called amblyopia.

The neurological basis of amblyopia has been discussed in Chap. 1. Changes in the anatomy of the lateral geniculate body have been demonstrated by von Noorden and in the macular thickness on optical coherence tomography by others [23, 24]. Reversal of these changes is unlikely in older individuals and hence the relevance of early management.

Broadly, the causes of amblyopia can be divided into abnormal binocular interaction and stimulus deprivation or a combination of the two. Amblyopia occurs during the sensitive period of visual maturation (initial 6–7 years) and thereafter the retinocortical pathways become resistant to abnormal visual inputs [21]. Earlier, longer, denser and more asymmetric the visual deprivation, greater the severity of amblyopia. Moreover, stimulus deprivation (e.g. congenital cataract) causes it to be more profound compared to abnormal binocular interaction (e.g. strabismus). Conditions in which both these factors act (e.g. unilateral congenital cataract) cause the densest amblyopia.

Salient features of an amblyopic eye are (1) subnormal near and distance visual acuity (2) subnormal colour vision, contrast and accommodation (3) fixation preference for the other eye (4) improvement in vision in mesopic (lesser light) conditions (5) crowding phenomenon (characters appear to run into one another) (6) eccentric fixation (7) absence of binocular summation i.e. visual acuity does not improve binocularly (8) slow and jerky pursuits (9) larger pupil and increased latency of reaction.

Labelling amblyopia as the cause of subnormal vision should only be done after excluding all other causes like VAO, irregular astigmatism, nystagmus, optic atrophy etc.

Visual outcomes after successful cataract surgery in children depend on the timely and adequate management of amblyopia. In order to treat amblyopia, the first step is to provide a sharp focussed image on to retina which is achieved after cataract surgery and appropriate refraction. In presence of asymmetry of vision between the two eyes, the next step is occluding the better eye to enforce fixation in the worse eye. Once this is achieved, the aim is to minimise aniseikonia and develop good, equal visual acuity in both eyes to stimulate fusion.

As discussed, amblyopia is profound in younger children, asymmetrical (or unilateral) cataract, denser cataract, delayed presentation and improper optical correction.

Occlusion of the sound eye is the mainstay of amblyopia management and is started soon after the glasses are prescribed. It is continued until normal, equal vision is achieved and the child is no longer at risk of redeveloping amblyopia. More profound the deprivation, longer and more intensive the treatment required [25]. Although various type of occlusion devices are available (Fig. 8.12), direct patching over the eye is the best as it does not permit peeking through the sides of glasses. Earlier full time occlusion was frequently prescribed, however this had poor compliance, unsatisfied parents and the risk of occlusion amblyopia in the

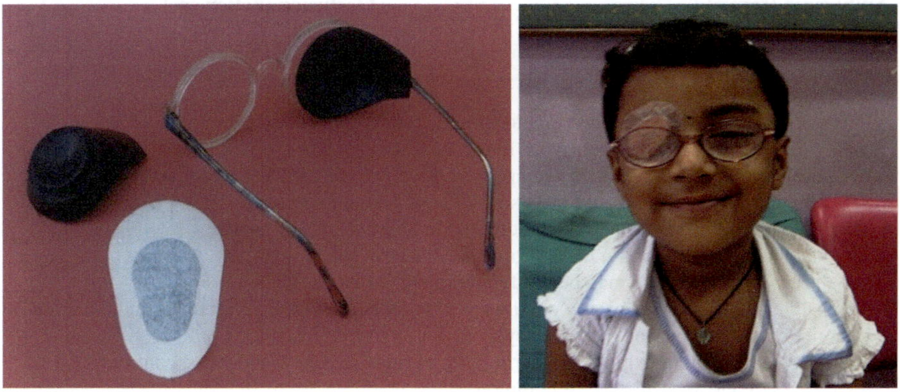

Fig. 8.12 Commonly used spectacle occluders (left) and child wearing a standard patch (right)

better eye. The usual occlusion regimens followed for infants and older children are listed in Tables 8.5 and 8.6 [3, 26–29]. Table 8.6 summarises the recommendations of the Pediatric Eye Disease Investigator Group (PEDIG). Though not specifically for amblyopia caused by developmental cataracts, it is understandable that regimens for same should only be stricter and prolonged. It should also be clear that these regimens are most effective when initiated in children below 5 years of age, with proper compliance and ensuring active use of the amblyopic eye during occlusion of the better eye.

Optical penalisation is practised sometimes in bilateral aphakia and pseudophakia, where occlusion cannot be employed due to bilaterality of the condition. In bilateral aphakia, eye with preferred fixation may be optically penalised by using the contact lens in this eye for 2–4 hours (h) lesser, compared to the amblyopic eye. Similarly, in pseudophakic children with a hyperopic refractive error, the dominant eye is left uncorrected for few hours each day, with the amblyopic eye fully corrected [30]. Glasses with appropriate correction in both eyes are used at other times.

Table 8.5 Occlusion regimen for infants after surgery for unilateral congenital cataract

Age (in months)	Occlusion (better eye)
<2	1–2 h/day
2–4	2–3 h/day
4–6	50% awake time
6–12	80% awake time

Though rare after unilateral cataract surgery, occlusion amblyopia (amblyopia of the better eye) due to treatment is a possibility in infants and preschool children. It is commoner after bilateral surgery and to prevent it the worse eye may also be occluded for a lesser duration depending on the age of the child. The physician and orthoptist should remain vigilant for it and should reconfirm if the parents have understood the occlusion regimen properly.

Table 8.6 Amblyopia management between 2 and 5 years of age (BCVA = best corrected visual acuity)

Amblyopia (severity)	Occlusion (better eye)
Moderate (BCVA 20/40–20/100)	2 h/day
Severe (BCVA 20/100–20/400)	6 h/day

Additional tips:

- During the period of occlusion the child should wear appropriate correction over the amblyopic eye and perform near work like reading or colouring.
- Children should be initially followed up every 4 weeks and then at 3 month intervals.
- Absence of improvement should raise suspicion of poor compliance.
- The duration of occlusion should be increased in absence of improvement.
- Pharmacological penalisation has no role after bilateral cataract surgery. Atropine penalisation of phakic eye may be tried in unilateral cases.
- Occlusion should be aggressively continued till there is no fixation preference and the child does not object to covering the better eye.
- After successful outcome gradual tapering of part time occlusion should be continued till 8–10 years of age as recurrence is common.

Presence of comorbidities like VAO and sensory nystagmus may limit visual outcomes. VAO needs to be managed surgically or by laser. In children with latent nystagmus, where occlusion exacerbates nystagmus, optical penalisation is particularly useful. This can be achieved by overcorrecting the hyperopia or by using lightly frosted glasses (prepared by painting neutral coloured nail enamel over the glass) in the better eye to reduce its vision by a line below the amblyopic eye [31]. It is also believed that the oscillopsia gradually improves if occlusion is continued [32]. Thus, optical penalisation and occlusion may need to be individualised in different situations while dealing with amblyopia associated with nystagmus.

Atropine penalisation is ineffective in children with bilateral aphakia or pseudophakia. Amongst pharmacological agents used for amblyopia management in older children, levodopa has been shown to be ineffective but results of citicoline have been promising [33–35]. Citicoline may be tried in children over 6 years of age who are not responding to conventional treatment or are having recurrence on tapering of occlusion.

Newer treatment modalities like digital amblyopia goggles are available, which can be programmed to occlude either eye for a predetermined duration each minute. They are unlikely to be popular in active children due to their cost and frequent breakage [31]. Use of dichoptic glasses while playing specialised video games for binocular visual stimulation is the newest promising treatment regimen [36].

Though we do not recommend pleoptics or office exercises (like CAM stimulator or Haidinger's brushes) to stimulate the macula in other types of amblyopia, we do feel they have a role in dense stimulus deprivation amblyopia caused by congenital cataracts [37, 38]. Moreover, they have additional benefit in bilateral amblyopia where occlusion is equivocal and when they are helpful in reducing the missed appointments [31, 39]. Binocular fixation preference in younger children and visual acuity in older children should be closely monitored to assess the response to amblyopia therapy and also to detect occlusion amblyopia early. Fixation preference as detailed in Chap. 3, is representative of the visual acuity. In presence of strabismus, ocular alignment should be considered.

As the vision improves, efforts to assess and improve binocular functions must be made. Achieving near-normal binocular single vision (BSV) would be the ultimate aim of management. Binocular summation (binocular vision better than uniocular), appreciation of physiological diplopia and correct response on Worth Four Dot Test (WFDT) can be used to ascertain the presence of BSV. Binocular vision is graded by responses on synoptophore and stereopsis is quantified by tests like Random Dot or Titmus Stereo. An expert orthoptist may use synoptophore, prisms or other means to reinforce binocular vision in children who have a good visual recovery with borderline binocularity.

Thus early surgery, optimal optical rehabilitation and amblyopia management are equally important for successful outcome of pediatric cataracts.

8.7 Comorbid Conditions

Presence of comorbid conditions like strabismus, nystagmus or searching movements are prognostic for poor outcome. While nystagmus can usually be attributed to other causes, strabismus and searching eye movements indicate a longer duration of visual deprivation. Similarly, co-existing anatomical abnormalities like coloboma, aniridia, microphthalmia or microcornea have sub-optimal outcomes. Presence of intraocular inflammation due to uveitis or following trauma predicts a long recovery course.

The presence of systemic involvement (e.g. Rubella or Down syndrome) severely compromises the management and the outcome.

8.8 Considering Refractive Procedures

An accurate biometric analysis, meticulous calculations and selection of appropriate IOL power help in achieving age-appropriate refractive error after cataract surgery in children. But in spite of all advances, in some cases, significant refractive error usually high myopia or astigmatism does occur. Refractive surprises are also commoner in children. Such children are best managed initially with contact lenses, however, if compliance is an issue a definitive surgery may be considered. Laser in situ keratomileusis (LASIK) is the most accurate method for correction, performed preferably at adolescence, after the refractive error has stabilised. Lens-based procedures, such as IOL exchange or piggyback lens implantation are alternatives [40]. They have been considered in Chap. 6.

8.9 Parent and Child Counselling

Untreated or partially treated pediatric cataracts lead to poor vision, which has a detrimental effect on child's education, occupation, and socio-economic status for life. Parental counselling in pediatric cataract management is essential and should begin at the time of surgical planning. The visual prognosis depending on the individual case should be discussed with the parents. The need for regular and multiple post-operative follow-ups, with adequate focus on the use of glasses and amblyopia therapy has to be clearly explained to parents. Possibility of second or third surgery as and when required in view of aphakia, strabismus, visual axis opacification, secondary glaucoma etc. is also an important aspect of parental counselling. However, all this should be done with empathy and care so that parents are not demotivated or discouraged to attempt for good visual outcomes.

8.10 Low Vision Rehabilitation

Children who undergo delayed surgery do not have a satisfactory visual recovery even after sincere rehabilitative measures. On the other hand, despite timely correction, optical rehabilitation and amblyopia management, some children may have suboptimal outcomes. Presence of nystagmus, poor fixation and strabismus indicate poorer visual prognosis. Visual potential can be enhanced in such children with the help of low vision rehabilitation team [28]. They play an important role in training these children according to their disability, helping them to lead a near-normal daily life and attain education. This is achieved by completely exploiting the remaining visual functions in conjunction with all other senses to achieve an optimum quality of life. Increasing the ambient light, allowing the children to sit closer to the blackboard in classes and increasing the font size of text are some simple environmental modification measures that help [41]. Aids for near vision are introduced when the reduction of the distance between the object and the eye does not allow the necessary range of visual function, or when the accommodative effort is too large. For aphakic or pseudophakic children with low vision (visual acuity is 20/70 or poorer in the better-seeing eye, which cannot be corrected or improved with regular eyeglasses), low vision devices based on their practical needs and utility can be prescribed.

Some of the most useful low vision devices based on school needs include telescope, hand magnifier, stand magnifier, digital devices with zoom-in function, contrast-enhancing devices and other non-optical devices [40] (Fig. 8.13).

Special schools for visual rehabilitation and education of visually impaired children have been established by the government, non-governmental organisations and private foundations. Children who are unable to manage in normal schools should be guided to these special schools in the locality, by the treating physician. Community participation is equally vital to mitigate the magnitude of their visual handicap. A responsible, gentle and caring approach of health workers and caregivers will be most effective in helping these children adjust to daily life activities [42]. At the same time, development of cost-effective, efficient and safe navigation systems for indoor and outdoor activities can help these children become more independent and enjoy a better quality of life [43].

True objective of pediatric cataract management is the integration of these children into the mainstream. The road is long and challenging but extremely rewarding.

8.11 Summary

- Regular follow-up and optimum visual restoration following cataract surgery are as imperative as surgery.
- Frequently changing refractive error, visual axis opacification and amblyopia are major challenges.
- Prescription of appropriate glasses or contact lens along with occlusion of better eye are the essential steps of visual restoration.

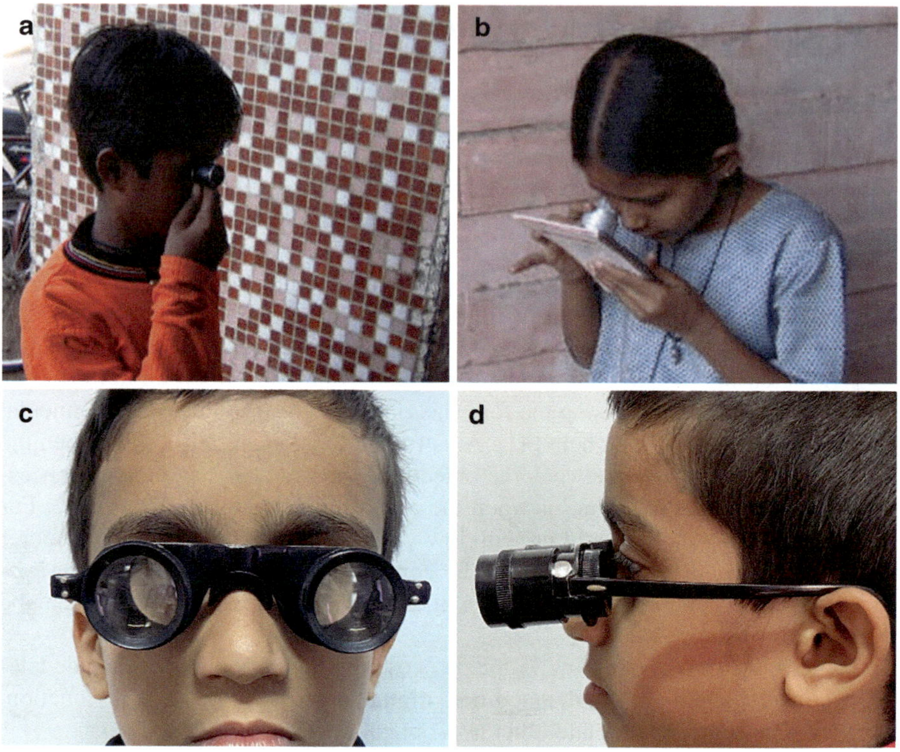

Fig. 8.13 Optical low vision devices (**a**) Handheld telescope, (**b**) Handheld magnifier, (**c** and **d**) Spectacle telescope. Different spectacles are required for distance and near. A headband may be used to reduce the weight on nose-bridge

- Children with untreatable low vision should be helped with the low vision aids to achieve maximum from their limited visual potential.
- A comprehensive approach, with cooperation between parents, surgeon, ophthalmic assistants and teachers is required to ensure successful rehabilitation of these children.

Multiple Choice Questions

1. Parameters to be evaluated on each follow up of a case operated for pediatric cataract:
   (a) Refraction, intraocular pressure and visual axis opacification
   (b) Corneal clarity, anterior chamber depth and IOL position
   (c) Conjunctival changes, corneal wounds and AC reaction
   (d) Vitreous opacities, axial length and keratometry

   Answer: *(a) Refraction, intraocular pressure and visual axis opacification*. All other factors are also important and need to be evaluated only in the first few follow-ups after surgery. However, refraction, IOP and VAO are 3 prime factors that may be expected to get deranged till later ages and require longer periods of follow-up.

2. A child of 1.5 years operated for cataract in both eyes. Her retinoscopy is +4 dioptre sphere (DS) post-operatively. Which of the following is the correct prescription for her?
   (a) +4 DS
   (b) +3 DS with near add of +2DS
   (c) +4 DS with near add of +1 DS
   (d) +5 DS

   Answer: *(d) +5DS*. Below 2 years of age near dominant glasses are prescribed. Bifocals are prescribed in older children.

3. Children who are left aphakic after cataract surgery should be prescribed glasses at which follow up:
   (a) After suture removal at 6 weeks
   (b) 4 weeks after suture removal
   (c) At 2 weeks post-operatively
   (d) Once the keratometry stabilises

   Answer: *(c) At 2 weeks post-operatively*. In children with aphakia, glasses should be prescribed as early as possible. Aphakic glasses may be given at the time of discharge after surgery or latest by 2 weeks to minimise amblyopia and allow age-related visual development.

4. While counselling the parents for cataract surgery of their child, which is the *least* important factor to be discussed with them:
   (a) Need of regular follow-ups
   (b) Need of post-operative use of glasses/contact lenses
   (c) May require a second surgery for clearing the visual axis
   (d) Manner of IOL power calculation and the type of IOL being implanted

   Answer: *(d) Manner of IOL power calculation and the type of IOL being implanted*. Though even this should be told to parents, it is more of the surgeons' responsibility to calculate the suitable IOL power according to age and the type of IOL suitable for that particular patient. Such information may sometimes confuse the parents. Other issues must be discussed with the parents as they form a vital part of visual rehabilitation after surgery.

5. Which of the following is NOT a predisposing factor for visual axis obscuration:
   (a) 3 mm capsulotomy
   (b) IOL implanted in the bag
   (c) Traumatic cataract
   (d) Child with rubella cataract

Answer: *(b) IOL implanted in the bag*. In the bag IOL implantation with posterior optic capture minimises the risk of VAO.

6. Which is the correct sequence of management after surgery for traumatic cataract in a 6-year old with intermittent exotropia. The child had sustained trauma 1 year back.
   (a) Refractive correction—occlusion of better eye—strengthening fusion—strabismus surgery.
   (b) Strabismus surgery—refractive correction—occlusion of better eye—strengthening fusion.
   (c) Occlusion of better eye–refractive correction–strengthening fusion–strabismus surgery.
   (d) Refractive correction–strabismus surgery–occlusion of better eye–strengthening fusion.

Answer: *(a) Refractive correction–occlusion of better eye–strengthening fusion–strabismus surgery.* Refractive correction should be the first step followed by amblyopia management by occlusion of the better eye. Intermittency of deviation shows that the child has binocularity, which can be improved by exercises. The child may be able to control the deviation well and not require surgery after improvement.

References

1. Anstice NS, Thompson B. The measurement of visual acuity in children: an evidence-based update. Clin Exp Optom. 2014;97(1):3–11.
2. Wilson ME, Trivedi RH. Pediatric cataract surgery techniques, complications, and management. Philadelphia, PA: Lippincott Williams & Wilkins; 2014. p. 303–6.
3. McClatchey SK, Parks MM. Theoretic refractive changes after lens implantation in childhood. Ophthalmology. 1997;104(11):1744–51.
4. Enyedi LB, Peterseim MW, Freedman SF, Buckley EG. Refractive changes after pediatric intraocular lens implantation. Am J Ophthalmol. 1998;126:772–8.
5. Ganesh S, Gupta R, Sethi S, Gurung C, Mehta R. Myopic shift after intraocular lens implantation in children less than two years of age. Nepal J Ophthalmol. 2018;10(19):11–5.
6. Sainani A. Special considerations for prescription of glasses in children. J Clin Ophthalmol Res. 2013;1:169–73.
7. Repka MX. Visual rehabilitation in pediatric aphakia. In: Nucci P, editor. Pediatric cataract. Developments in ophthalmology, vol. 57. Basel: Karger; 2016. p. 49–68.
8. Wilson ME Jr, Bartholomew LR, Trivedi RH. Pediatric cataract surgery and intraocular lens implantation: practice styles and preferences of the 2001 ASCRS and AAPOS memberships. J Cataract Refract Surg. 2003;29:1811–20.
9. Baradaran-Rafii A, Shirzadeh E, Eslani M, Akbari M. Optical correction of aphakia in children. J Ophthalmic Vis Res. 2014;9(1):71–82.
10. Lambert SR, Lynn MJ, et al. Infant Aphakia Treatment Study Group; A randomized clinical trial comparing contact lens to intraocular lens correction of monocular aphakia during infancy: HOTV optotype acuity at age 4.5 years and clinical findings at age 5 years. The Infant Aphakia Treatment Study (IATS). JAMA Ophthalmol. 2014;132:676–82.

11. Neely DE, Plager DA, Borger SM, et al. Accuracy of intraocular lens calculations in infants and children undergoing cataract surgery. J AAPOS. 2005;9:160–5.
12. Shenoy BH, Mittal V, Gupta A, Sachdeva V, Kekunnaya R. Refractive outcomes and prediction error following secondary intraocular lens implantation in children: a decade-long analysis. Br J Ophthalmol. 2013;97(12):1516–9.
13. Kekunnaya R, Gupta A, Sachdeva V, Rao HL, Vaddavalli PK, Om Prakash V. Accuracy of intraocular lens power calculation formulae in children less than two years. Am J Ophthalmol. 2012;154(1):13–9.
14. VanderVeen DK, Trivedi RH, Nizam A, et al. Predictability of intraocular lens power calculation formulae in infantile eyes with unilateral congenital cataract: results from the Infant Aphakia Treatment Study. Am J Ophthalmol. 2013;156:1252–60.
15. Dahan E, Drusedau MU. Choice of lens and dioptric power in pediatric pseudophakia. J Cataract Refract Surg. 1997;23:618–23.
16. O'Keefe M, Mulvihill A, Yeoh PL. Visual outcome and complications of bilateral intraocular lens implantation in children. J Cataract Refract Surg. 2000;26:1758–64.
17. Kohnen T, Fabian E, Gerl R, Hunold W, Hütz W, Strobel J, et al. Optic edge design as long-term factor for posterior capsular opacification rates. Ophthalmology. 2008;115:1308–14.
18. Trivedi RH, Wilson ME, Bartholomew LR, Lal G, Peterseim MM. Opacification of the visual axis after cataract surgery and single acrylic intraocular lens implantation in the first year of life. J AAPOS. 2004;8:156–64.
19. Von Noorden GK. Binocular vision and ocular motility. Mosby-Year Book Inc: St Louis, MO; 1990.
20. Agrawal S, Singh N, Singh V. Non surgical treatment of Strabismus. In: Agrawal S, editor. Strabismus for every ophthalmologist. 1st ed. Singapore: Springer; 2019. p. 105–7.
21. Birch EE, Cheng C, Stager DR Jr, Felius J. Visual acuity development after the implantation of unilateral intraocular lenses in infants and young children. J AAPOS. 2005;9:527–32.
22. Von Noorden GK, Campos EC. Binocular vision and ocular motility. 6th ed. St. Louis: Mosby; 2002. p. 246–86. Chapter 14: Amblyopia
23. Yen MY, Cheng CY, Wang AG. Retinal nerve fiber layer thickness in unilateral amblyopia. Invest Ophthalmol Vis Sci. 2004;45(7):2224–30.
24. Agrawal S, Singh V, Singhal V. Cross sectional study of macular thickness variations in unilateral amblyopia. J Clin Ophthalmol Res. 2014;2(1):15–7.
25. Singh V, Agrawal S. Visual functions in amblyopia as determinants of response to treatment. J Pediatr Ophthalmol Strabismus. 2013;50(6):348–54.
26. Scheiman MM, Hertle RW, Beck RW, et al., Pediatric Eye Disease Investigator Group. Randomized trial of treatment of amblyopia in children aged 7 to 17 years. Arch Ophthalmol. 2005;123(4):437–47.
27. Repka MX, Beck RW, Holmes JM, et al., Pediatric Eye Disease Investigator Group. A randomized trial of patching regimens for treatment of moderate amblyopia in children. Arch Ophthalmol. 2003;121(5):603–11.
28. Holmes JM, Kraker RT, Beck RW, et al., Pediatric Eye Disease Investigator Group. A randomized trial of prescribed patching regimens for treatment of severe amblyopia in children. Ophthalmology. 2003;110(11):2075–87.
29. Vagge A, Nelson LB. Amblyopia update: new treatments. Curr Opin Ophthalmol. 2016;27:380–6.
30. Kim DH, Kim JH, Kim SJ, et al. Long-term results of bilateral congenital cataract treated with early cataract surgery, aphakic glasses and secondary IOL implantation. Acta Ophthalmol. 2012;90:231–6.
31. Agrawal S, Singh N, Singh V. Chapter 6: Non surgical treatment of strabismus. In: Strabismus for every ophthalmologist. 1st ed. Singapore: Springer; 2019. p. 101–14.
32. Von Noorden GK, Campos EC. Binocular vision and ocular motility. 6th ed. St. Louis: Mosby; 2002. p. 537–53. Chapter 24: Principles of nonsurgical treatment

33. Repka MX, Kraker RT, Dean TW, et al. Pediatric Eye Disease Investigator Group. A randomized trial of levodopa as treatment for residual amblyopia in older children. Ophthalmology. 2015;122:874–81.
34. Fresina M, Dickmann A, Salerni A, et al. Effect of oral CDP-choline on visual function in young amblyopic patients. Graefes Arch Clin Exp Ophthalmol. 2008;246:143–50.
35. Pawar PV, Mumbare SS, Patil MS, et al. Effectivemenss of the addition of citicoline to patching in the treatment of amblyopia around visual maturity: a randomized controlled trial. Indian J Ophthalmol. 2014;62:124–9.
36. Hess RF, Mansouri B, Thompson B. A new binocular approach to the treatment of amblyopia in adults well beyond the critical period of visual development. Restor Neurol Neurosci. 2010;28:793–802.
37. Verma A, Singh D. Rehabilitation and management of pseudophakic amblyopia in cases of unilateral congenital cataract by active vision therapy. Ann Ophthalmol. 2007;39:284–90.
38. Sahu CL, Muralidhar R, Ramamurthy D. A preliminary study on the treatment of amblyopia with Haidinger's brushes. J Clin Ophthalmol Res. 2020;8:10–3.
39. Huang HM, Kuo HK, Fang PC, Lin HF, Lin PW, Lin SA. The effects of CAM vision stimulator for bilateral amblyopia of different etiologies. Chang Gung Med J. 2008;31(6):592–8.
40. Abdelghany AA, Alio JL. Surgical options for correction of refractive error following cataract surgery. Eye Vis (Lond). 2014;1:2.
41. Minto H, Butt IA. Low vision devices and training. Community Eye Health. 2004;17(49):6–7.
42. Stevens S. Assisting the blind and visually impaired: guidelines for eye health workers and other helpers. Community Eye Health. 2003;16(45):7–9.
43. Real S, Araujo A. Navigation systems for the blind and visually impaired: past work, challenges, and open problems. Sensors (Basel). 2019;19(15):3404.

GPSR Compliance

The European Union's (EU) General Product Safety Regulation (GPSR) is a set of rules that requires consumer products to be safe and our obligations to ensure this.

If you have any concerns about our products, you can contact us on ProductSafety@springernature.com

In case Publisher is established outside the EU, the EU authorized representative is:

Springer Nature Customer Service Center GmbH
Europaplatz 3
69115 Heidelberg, Germany

Batch number: 10726135

Printed by Printforce, the Netherlands